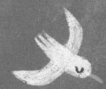

BIBLE STORIES
for KIDS

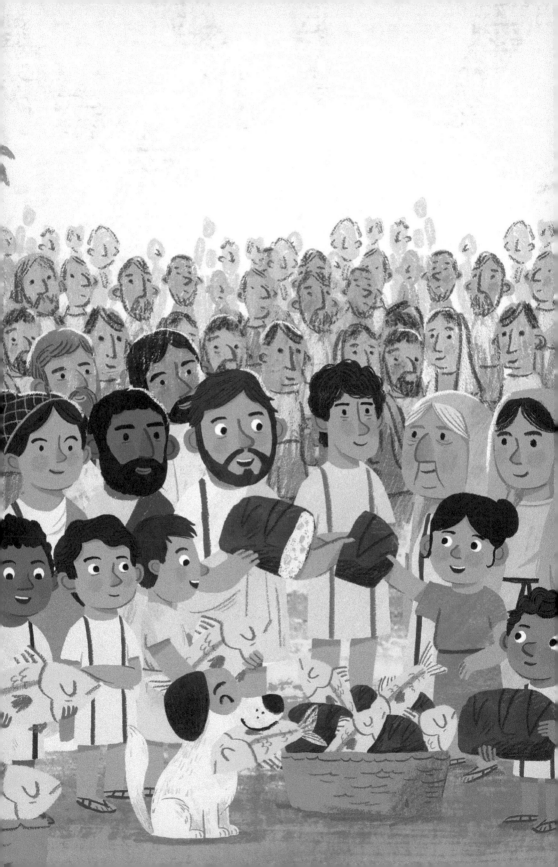

BIBLE STORIES
for KIDS

40 Essential Stories to Grow in God's Love

BONNIE RICKNER JENSEN

Illustrations by Patrick Corrigan

ROCKRIDGE
PRESS

For general information on our other products and services or to obtain technical support, please contact our Customer Care Department within the United States at (866) 744-2665, or outside the United States at (510) 253-0500.

Rockridge Press publishes its books in a variety of electronic and print formats. Some content that appears in print may not be available in electronic books, and vice versa.

Interior and Cover Designer: Angie Chiu
Art Producer: Hannah Dickerson
Editor: Laura Apperson
Production Editor: Ruth Sakata Corley
Production Manager: Jose Olivera

Illustrations © 2021 Patrick Corrigan

Scripture taken from the International Children's Bible®. Copyright © 1986, 1988, 1999 by Thomas Nelson. Used by permission. All rights reserved.

ISBN: Print 978-1-64876-942-9
eBook 978-1-64876-274-1
R0

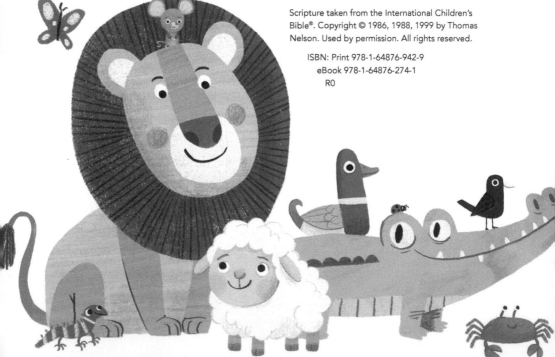

CONTENTS

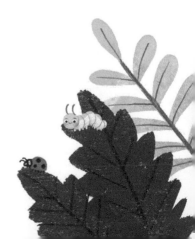

THE NEW TESTAMENT

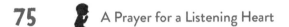

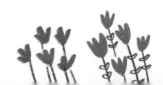

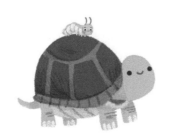
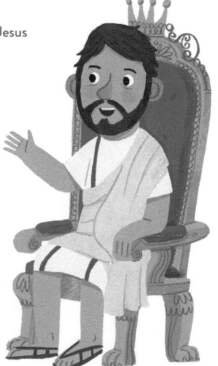

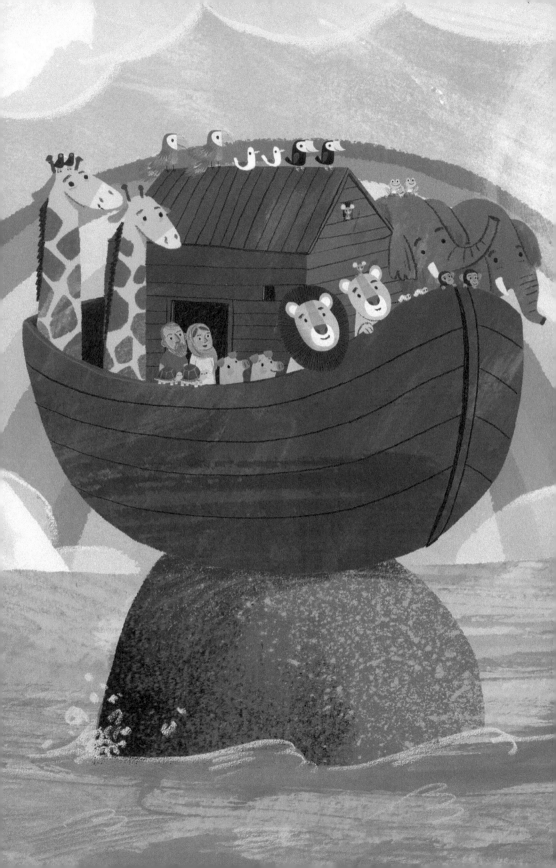

A NOTE FOR PARENTS

This book is written to lead a child's heart to the deep, daring love of our perfect, powerful God. Children will see themselves in these pages and understand that God chooses the small, the weak, and even those who are afraid, to do great and mighty things in the world. With scripture references and questions designed to help children talk about God's Word—and how it applies to their own experiences and feelings—this book is a priceless addition to any home library. Focused on God's goodness, *Bible Stories for Kids* gives children confidence in knowing they're secure in His hands and held by His incredible *forever* love for them.

THE OLD TESTAMENT

GOD'S CREATION, OUR HOME

GENESIS 1–2

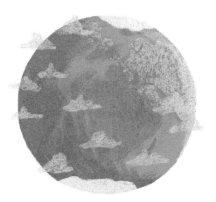

In the beginning, God painted the sky and sculpted the earth. The earth was dark. No life was found. Then came a powerful, pleasing sound. God's voice thundered, *"Let there be light!"* And so there was! It was good, like *all* our loving God does. He called the light "day" and the darkness "night."

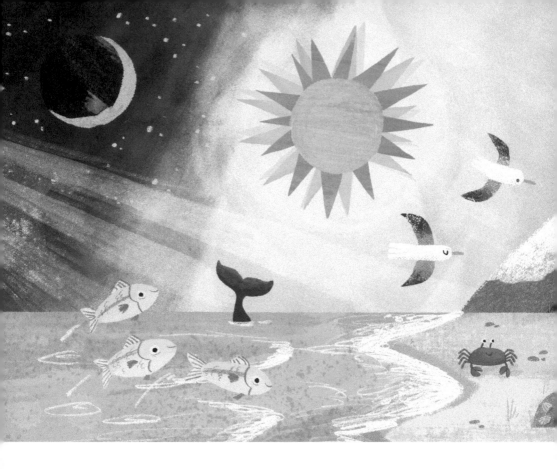

God drew lines around the oceans. He left land
in perfect shapes and places. Trees and plants
sprang up everywhere. Fruit holding seeds hung
from the trees. God put great lights in the sky. He
made a bright yellow sun and a milky white moon.
He scattered sparkling jewels over the bedtime
sky. He called them "stars." God filled the seas with
swimming creatures. He decorated the sky with
soaring birds.

God had fun creating animals. Some were wild!
Others were tame. He stretched the giraffe's neck.

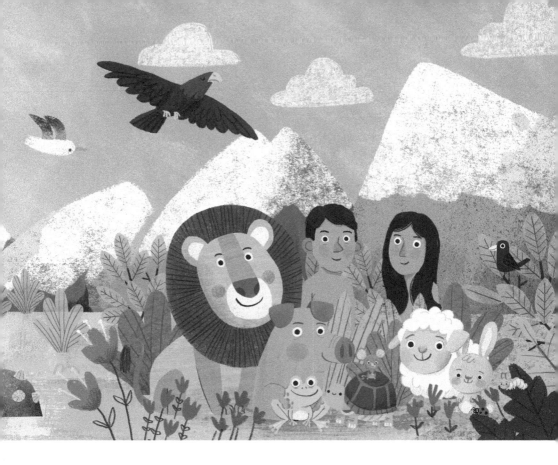

He fluffed the lion's mane. The zebra got stripes. The leopard got spots. The bunny's tail puffed. And the chipmunk's cheeks were made to be stuffed!

God saved His favorite for last. He made the first people. He loved them more than *anything* in the whole universe. He still does. He created people in His own image! Their names were Adam and Eve.

Whew! God's creation took six days to finish. On day seven, God rested.

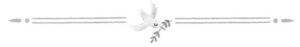

The sky, the earth and all that filled them were finished. On the seventh day He rested from all His work. God blessed the seventh day and made it a holy day.

Genesis 2:1–3

*Why do you think God made the day of rest **holy**? Sunday is a lazy day for lots of families. When people rest, that's often when they're able to most clearly understand God and His loving messages.*

A PRAYER OF APPRECIATION FOR GOD'S CREATION

Dear God,

Thank You for creating the earth, the sky, the sea, and me. I'll always put my trust in You—Your perfect love's in *all* You do!

A BEAUTIFUL GARDEN WITH A SLY SNAKE

GENESIS 3

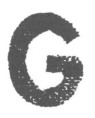od gave Adam and Eve a perfect place to live. He planted a beautiful garden in a land called Eden. God told them to enjoy every good thing growing in the garden, except He warned them not to taste the fruit hanging from *one* tree. It was a simple rule. But a sly snake slithered in the garden. The snake didn't like God *or* His rules. It came to trick Adam and Eve into disobeying. It wanted them to forget God's love long enough to make a terrible mistake.

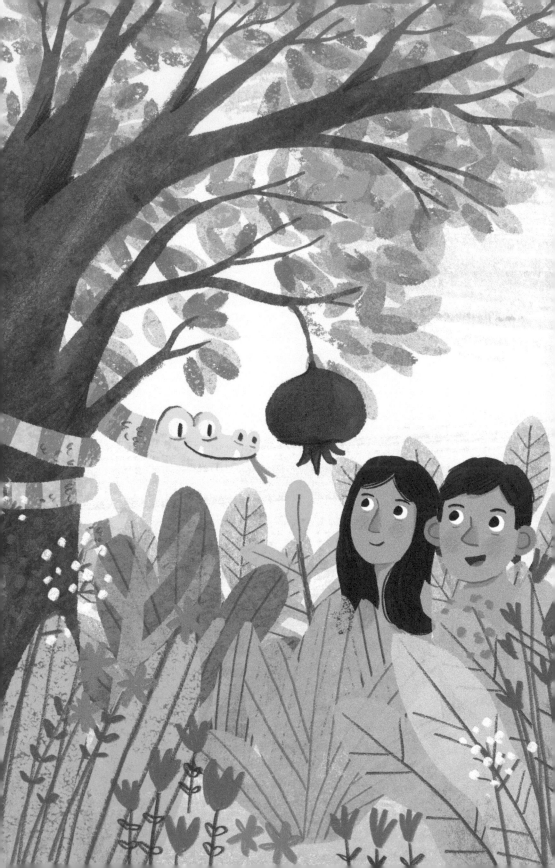

The snake hissed. It whispered to Eve, "Eat from the *one* tree. Then you'll see things as God does! If God loves you, wouldn't He want you to become wise?" Adam and Eve believed the sneaky snake's lie. They took a bite of the fruit from the *one* tree. Suddenly, everything changed. One lie allowed an awful thing to enter the world. **Sin** found its way into the hearts of Adam and Eve. Suddenly they felt sad and afraid.

The perfect life God created for them was now imperfect. They walked out of the garden to begin their new journey. God told them He would watch over them. He loved them as much as ever! But they had to leave their perfect home. God had a plan to squash sin and the lies it brought. A mistake can't keep God's great big love from reaching out. It *never* will.

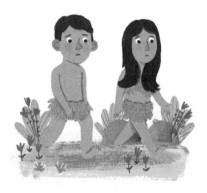

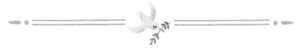

Nothing can separate us from the love God has for us. Not death, not life, not angels, not ruling spirits, nothing now, nothing in the future, no powers, nothing above us, nothing below us, or anything else in the whole world will ever be able to separate us from the love of God.

Romans 8:38

? Do you feel bad when you forget to follow a rule? It's okay to think about how you might do better next time around. But don't keep feeling badly when you do a bad thing. God is all-forgiving!

NOAH AND THE AMAZING ARK

GENESIS 6–9

After God's creation, many people filled the earth. Sadly, most forgot about God's never-ending love. They ignored what was good and right. It hurt God's heart to see them hurt one another. It hurt to see them destroy their beautiful earthly home.

God found one man who turned His frown upside down! The man's name was Noah. Noah loved to pray. That means he loved talking to God. Noah was a good listener with a good heart. God warned Noah of a coming flood. The earth was going to get a fresh start.

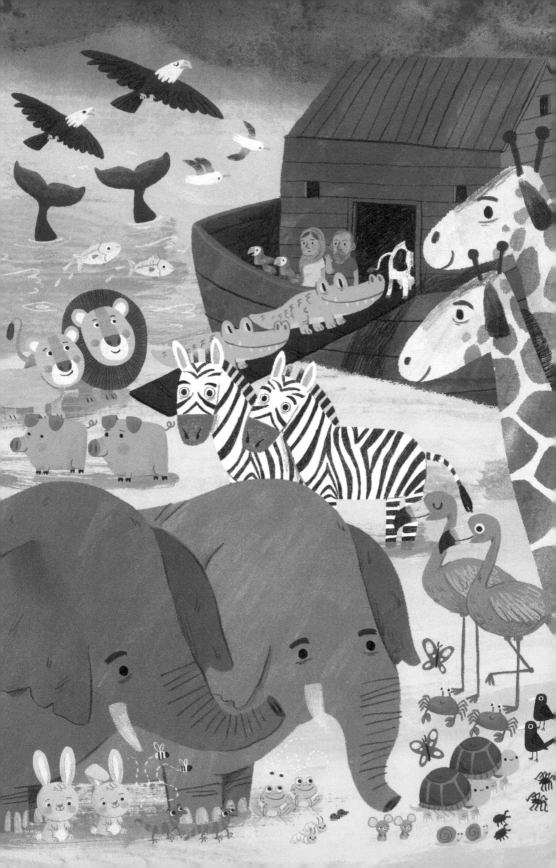

God gave Noah an important assignment. He told him to build an **ark**. The gigantic boat would save Noah's family. God planned to send two of *every* kind of animal to join them. There would be animals that roared, soared, hopped, clopped, crawled, screeched, squawked, and climbed!

Noah did as God said. He built the ark. The ark had stalls for cows and sheep. It had bunks for skunks to curl up and sleep. It stored food for everyone to eat. Finally, the rainstorm started. For forty days and nights the drops didn't stop! The flood flowed over the mountaintops. God watched and protected the ark. At the perfect time, the water dried up. The ark teetered on the tip of Mount Ararat. Sunbeams reached through the clouds. The beams painted a rainbow across the sky. God put a promise inside every rainbow: *I love you, and I'll never flood the earth again.*

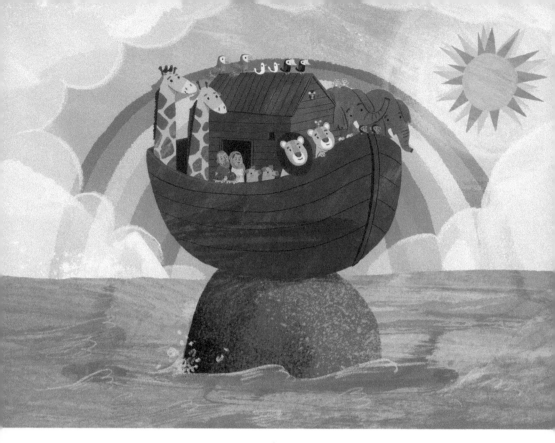

Floodwaters will never again destroy all life on the earth. When the rainbow appears in the clouds, I will see it. Then I will remember the agreement that continues forever.

Genesis 9:15–16

? *What do you think makes God smile? Pray to God that you might see the world through His eyes. Look around, and point out all God's beauty and blessings that surround you. His love is everywhere!*

A WIFE GIGGLES— HUBBY'S FAITH DOESN'T WIGGLE!

GENESIS 12–21

A braham served God with a *strong* **faith**. He obeyed God with a trusting heart. One night God spoke to Abraham under a clear, starry sky. He told Abraham to look up and count the stars. God wanted Abraham to see how big his family would be one day. It would outnumber the stars!

Time passed and Abraham became discouraged. He believed God's promise, but it was taking a long time for it to come true. He

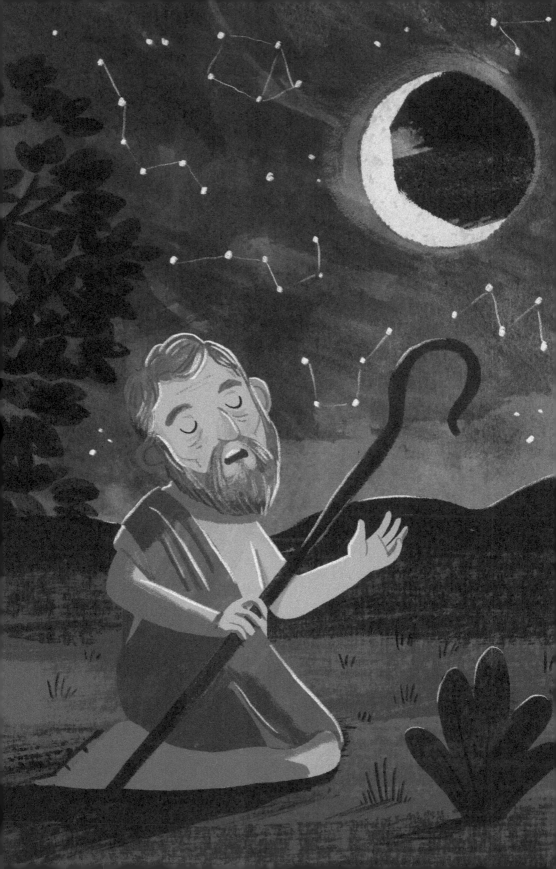

and his wife, Sarah, were almost 100 years old. They still didn't have a child! Sarah giggled at God's promise to give them a child. But Abraham's faith in God never wiggled.

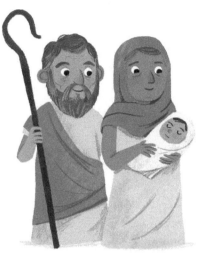

After a long and patient wait, Abraham and Sarah had a son. They named him Isaac, which means, "he laughs." All the giggling in Abraham's family was now because of God's goodness. When God's promises come true, faith muscles get bigger and stronger, too.

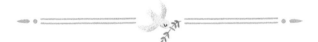

The Lord cared for Sarah as He had said.
He did for her what He had promised.

Genesis 21:1

❓ *When you have to wait for something, do you show patience? God knows the perfect timing for **everything**.*

FROM DREAMER TO RULER

GENESIS 37–45

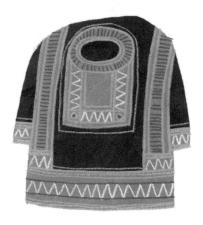

J acob had thirteen children—twelve sons and one daughter. He loved them all. But his young son Joseph had a special place in his heart. Jacob gave Joseph a fancy, ornamental long-sleeved robe. Joseph's brothers didn't like that one bit.

"Why does he get special clothing from dad?" they grumbled. They were jealous of their little brother. Joseph started telling his brothers about the dreams God gave him. That's when things got worse!

"In my dreams you bow down to me," Joseph told his brothers. Their jealousy soon turned to hate. They couldn't take another minute of Joseph being the "favorite." The angry brothers sold him as a servant. They lied and told Jacob he had died. They

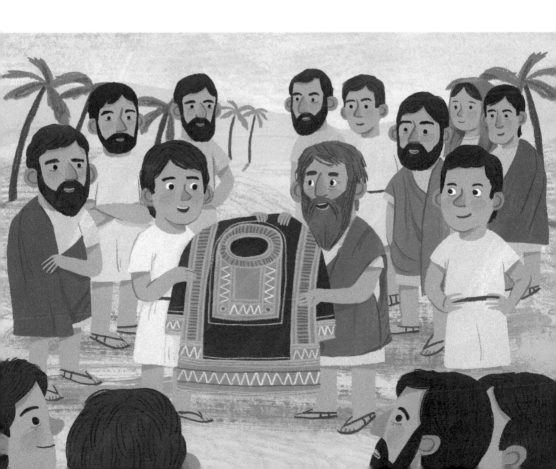

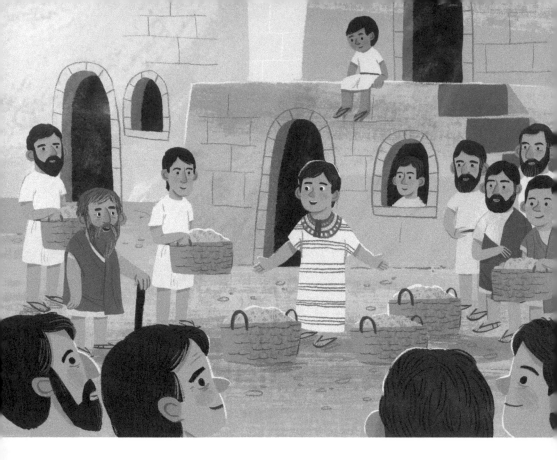

didn't know God's plan. God planned to take Joseph from being a servant to a powerful ruler.

Joseph trusted God. He didn't grumble while he scrubbed floors as a servant. He stayed positive when he was unjustly put in prison. When the king of Egypt needed a mighty ruler, he chose Joseph. The king knew God had given Joseph the gift of understanding dreams.

In time, Joseph's family had no food to eat. There was a **famine** in the land. The brothers came to Egypt hoping for help. God's love was in Joseph's heart. He forgave his brothers' meanness. He gave them everything they needed and more. That's the way God gives!

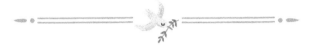

Joseph gave them wagons. And he gave them food for their trip. He gave each brother a change of clothes. Joseph also sent his father donkeys loaded with the best things from Egypt. They were loaded with grain, bread and other food.

Genesis 45:21–23

❓ *One of God's specialties is bringing about good things from the bad. He loves with all His heart. How do you keep a good attitude when things don't seem to be going so well? Can you think of something in your life you thought would be terrible but turned out to be a blessing?*

MIRACLES THROUGH MOSES

EXODUS 2–14

There once was a **pharaoh** in Egypt. The pharaoh was afraid of being overtaken by the Israelites. So he tried to keep their families from growing. It didn't work! God used two kind and caring nurses to help stop the pharaoh's ugly plan. One Israelite mother had a baby boy. She *knew* her baby was special. She knew as soon as she held him for the first time. She hid him from the pharaoh. Then she sent the baby down the river in a basket. This decision saved his life. The boy's name became Moses.

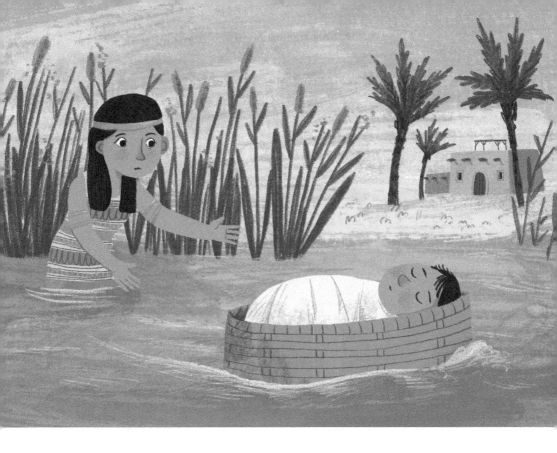

Moses grew up. He fled from Egypt for a while. One day God spoke to him from a burning bush! God's voice rumbled out of the flames. God told Moses to go back to Egypt. He told him to free the Israelite slaves. The slaves were treated cruelly. They were suffering. God heard His children crying. His love would turn everything around.

Moses wasn't sure he could do what God had asked. But God promised to make him brave and strong. God used the walking stick Moses carried. He used it to show the pharaoh He was real and mighty.

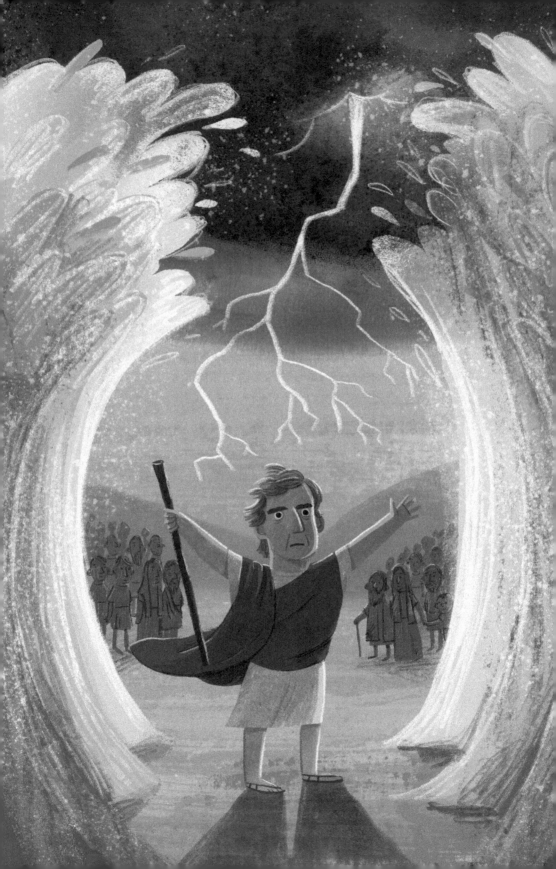

He used it to show He was there to get His people out of Egypt. The stick turned into a serpent! Then it turned back into a stick again! Moses held the stick up to the Red Sea. The sea parted and rose to the sky. Moses and his people walked safely between the towers of water! God's miraculous love saved His children.

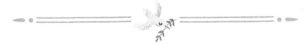

The Lord said, "I have seen the troubles my people have suffered in Egypt. And I have heard their cries when the Egyptian slave masters hurt them. I am concerned about their pain. I have come down to save them. I will bring them out of that land. I will lead them to a good land."

Exodus 3:7–8

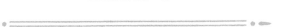

❓ *God is always creating ways to show His forever love for **you**. What are some ways you feel safe in God's care? Can you think of a moment you knew was God's doing that took you by surprise?*

THE TEN COMMANDMENTS

EXODUS 19–20

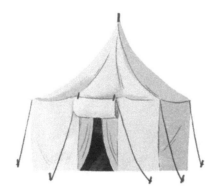

It had been three months since Moses led the Israelites out of Egypt. God had saved them from an angry pharaoh!

He was leading them to a **promised land**! On their way they camped at Mount Sinai. They built campfires. They raised tents.

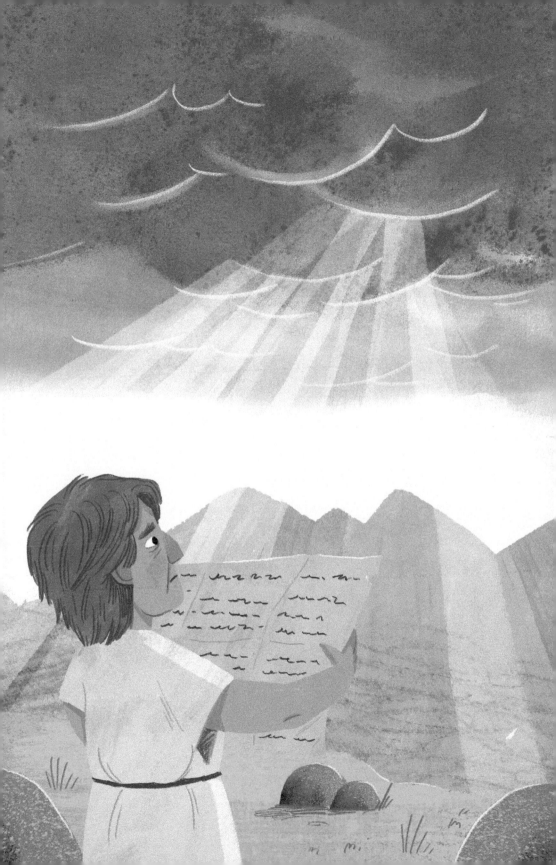

Then a loud rumble shook the mountain. God was calling for Moses!

God told Moses He was going to give His people ten rules. By obeying these rules, they'd show their love for Him. The people agreed to do what God asked. They knew God loved them very much.

Three days passed. Moses met God on the mountain to hear the **commandments**. God came down wrapped in a robe of dense clouds. Thunder rolled! Lightning flashed! *BANG! BOOM! CRASH! CLAP!* God's voice was loud. The ground shook. Moses listened *closely* to God's rules:

1) Follow only God. 2) Worship only God. 3) Be kind when using God's name. 4) Rest on the Lord's holy day. 5) Respect your parents. 6) Do not kill. 7) Do not steal. 8) Do not lie. 9) Be loyal to marriage promises. 10) Don't want what belongs to others.

We're children of God, too! These rules are for us to obey. God gave them because He loves us. He wants our lives to be filled with good things that come from His great love.

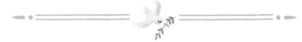

The Lord came down on the top of
Mount Sinai. Then He called Moses to
come up to the top of the mountain.

Exodus 19:20

? *You are a child of God. God's rules are for you, too. How does it make your heart feel when you break a rule of God? God loves you. He wants what is best for you!*

A PRAYER TO BEHAVE, DO RIGHT, AND BE BRAVE

Dear God,

Your commandments teach me what is good and how to live the way I should. Give me courage, make me strong, to do what's right and not what's wrong.

THE WALLS WILL FALL!

JOSHUA 5-6

Joshua was a brave warrior. God chose him to be the one to finally lead the Israelites into the promised land. It was lush land. It had good soil to grow lots of delicious food! God knew His people would be weary from their long journey. The promised land would feel like a nice, soft bed. It would feel like God's warm, gentle love.

The people had walked in the desert for forty years. They were ready to reach their wonderful land. But the city of Jericho stood in their way. Jericho had soaring walls and tall iron gates. The gates were locked up tight.

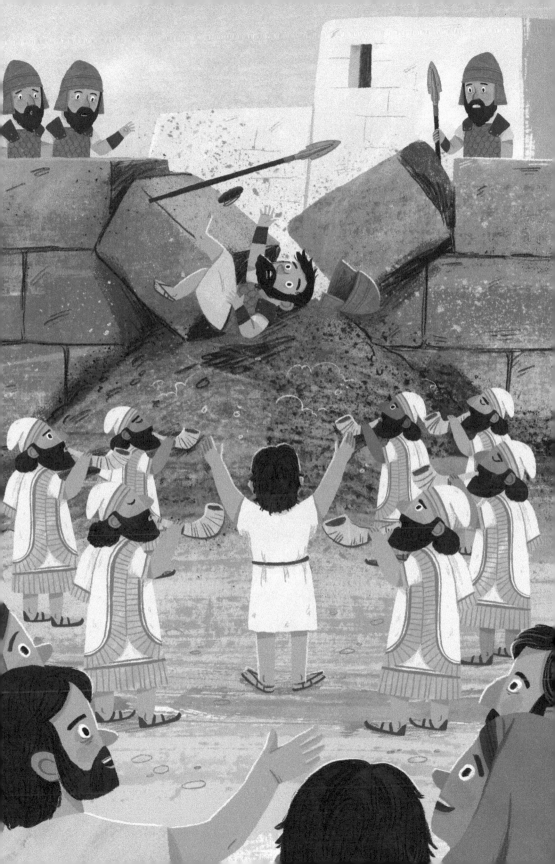

No one was let in or out. The people of Jericho knew Joshua was coming with all God's might!

Some of Joshua's army had weapons. But they didn't need them. God told Joshua they would march in! Each day, for six days, they marched around the city. On the seventh day they marched around the city *seven* times. They blew trumpets as they marched. They put their trust in God without a doubt. At Joshua's command they let out a *SHOUT*! The air filled with the sound of rumbles. The massive walls suddenly crumbled! The city of Jericho was out of their way. They entered their promised land, cheering *HOORAY*!

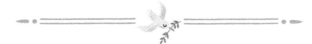

The Lord spoke to Joshua. He said,
"Look, I have given you Jericho, its king and
all its fighting men. The walls of the city will fall.
And the people will go straight into the city."
Joshua 6:2–5

? *Do you remember a time when you needed to be especially brave? Did you turn to God for help? Don't be afraid to ask! God will give you courage every time.*

DEBORAH AND HER DARING HEART

JUDGES 4–5

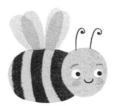

The name Deborah means "bee." The name perfectly fits this strong, gifted woman of God! Deborah was the fifth **judge** to serve the people of Israel. At the time, they were closing their ears to God's voice. They did things they'd been commanded not to do!

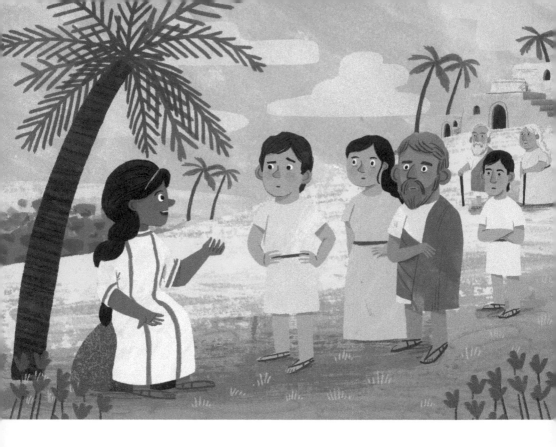

Deborah didn't have a courtroom. She sat at the base of a palm tree to give her rulings. This tree was known as the Palm of Deborah. From this spot she listened closely to God. God told her to talk to an army commander named Barak. She told Barak God would give him victory over Sisera. Sisera was a warrior who'd been bullying the Israelites for twenty years. Barak said to Deborah, "I'll go to battle if you go with me."

Deborah knew God would go ahead of them. So she went with Barak. God helped them defeat the cruel warrior. Sisera's bullying days were over. God's people then lived in peace for forty years. Deborah gave all the praise to God. She wrote a beautiful song for Him. She was a judge, prophetess, poet, and brave leader. She truly was as busy as a bee!

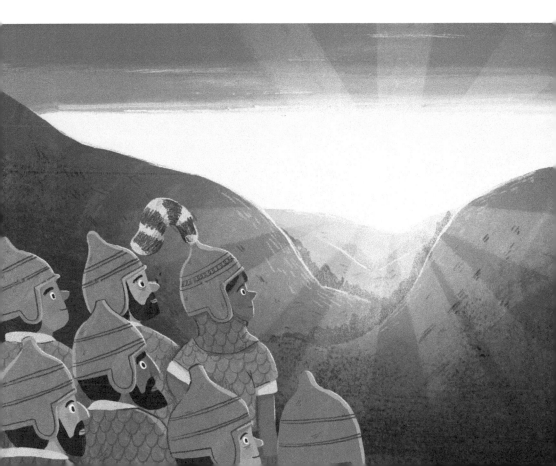

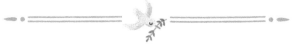

Barak said to Deborah,
"If you will not go with me, I won't go."

"Of course I will go with you," Deborah answered.
"But you will not get credit for the victory.
The Lord will let a woman defeat Sisera."

Judges 4:8–9

? *Deborah, the "busy bee," had the gifts of* **wisdom***, good judgment, and bravery! You, too, have gifts from God. What activities do you like to do when you want to get busy? What do you see as your greatest strengths?*

GOD CALLS EVEN THE SMALL

JUDGES 6-7

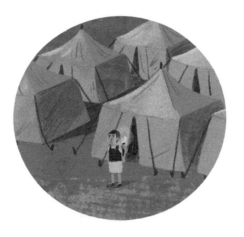

Gideon didn't feel strong or special. He belonged to the weakest group among God's people. He was not the strongest one in his family. But God sees strength in those who do not feel very brave. God sent an angel to Gideon. The angel said, "The Lord is with you. You are mighty!"

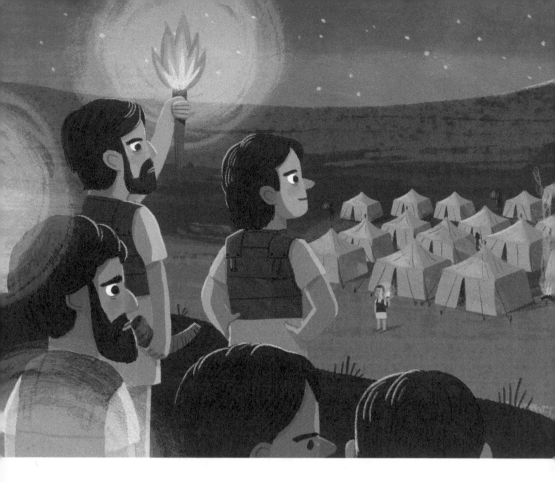

"Mighty?" Gideon responded. "You must have me
mixed up with someone else!" God didn't have anything mixed up. God doesn't make mistakes. God's
plan for Gideon was to free the Israelites. The people
of Midian were smashing their crops and stealing
their animals. With God by his side, Gideon did
just that. The Lord instructed Gideon to take only
300 men to battle. Their enemy was much greater in
number! Gideon and his men surrounded the enemy

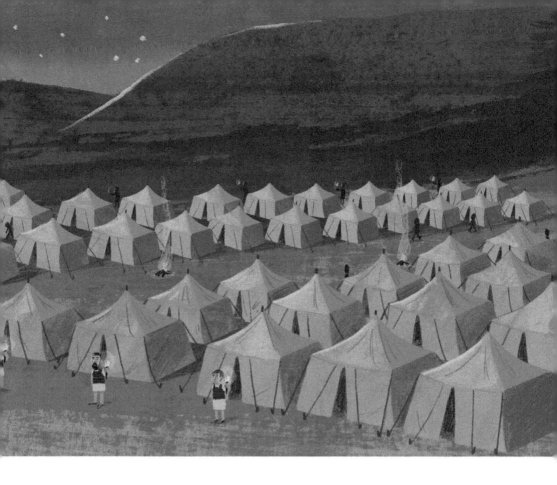

camp. They lifted torches in their left hands. They held trumpets in their right hands. They shouted, "For the Lord and for Gideon!"

The enemy thought thousands of men were with Gideon, not hundreds. So off they ran! It was God's perfect plan. God used Gideon for such an amazing feat. Everyone saw God's faithfulness. They realized *each* of His children is incredibly special.

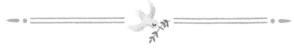

The Midianites came up and camped in the land. They brought their tents and their animals with them. They were like swarms of locusts! There were so many people and camels they could not be counted. These people came into the land to ruin it. So the Israelites cried out to the Lord for help.

Judges 6:5–6

We are wonderfully and marvelously made! Gideon was small in **stature** *but big in his belief in God. What do you feel are some of your best qualities? Share your gratitude. God loves to hear from you!*

A GOOD FRIEND
IS A GIFT
FROM GOD

RUTH 1–4

A young woman named Ruth and her **mother-in-law**, Naomi, were good friends. Ruth loved Naomi as her own mother. Naomi loved Ruth like a daughter. They lived in a place called Moab. Trouble came to their lives. Their husbands died. Ruth promised she would never leave Naomi's side. Naomi tried to talk Ruth into living in a different land. She wanted Ruth to think about herself. She wanted what was best for Ruth. But Ruth stayed by Naomi's side. She would not leave!

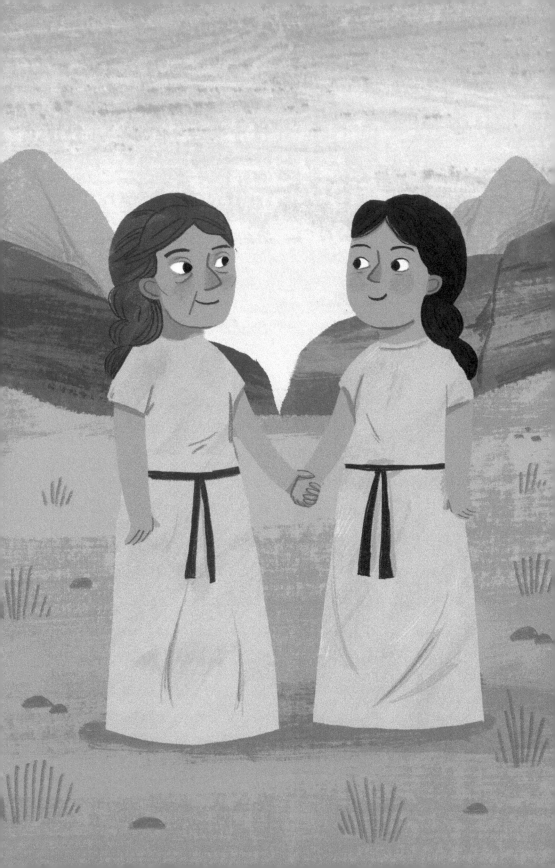

The two women went to Bethlehem together. Boaz, a kind and **generous** man, heard how good Ruth was to Naomi. He married Ruth. She gave birth to a son. Naomi's heart was filled with excitement and **joy**! She held her baby grandson. She couldn't stop smiling. God brought them more happiness than they ever imagined possible. They had felt sad for so long. Now, God gave them a new family.

Through the gift of a good friendship, God gave Ruth and Naomi lots of blessings. The two made friends with many other women in their new home. Sometimes God shows His heart through friends. God's love *never* leaves.

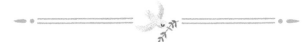

The women told Naomi, "Praise the Lord Who gave you this grandson. He will give you new life. And he will take care of you in your old age. This happened because of your daughter-in-law. She loves you."

Ruth 4:14–15

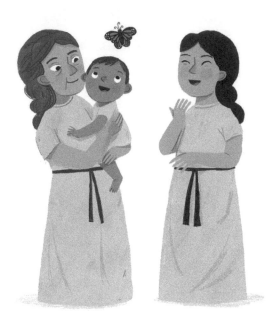

? *A best friend is someone who is very good at being thoughtful! (God is the best friend* **anyone** *could have.) Do you have a friend you're especially thankful for? Say a prayer of appreciation.*

A PRAYER OF FRIENDSHIP AND FAITHFULNESS

Dear God,

You've given me gifts that are one of a kind. A better friend I'll never find. You know my heart and silent prayers. Your faithful love is everywhere.

HANNAH'S HOPE

1 SAMUEL 1–2

Hannah was a woman who loved God. She wanted to have children. She wanted this more than anything else in the world. She worshiped God purely. She loved Him with her whole heart. She prayed for a child with eager desire! It started to feel like a long, long time to wait. Hannah became more and more sad. It seemed God wasn't listening. But Hannah kept hoping. And God heard *every* word Hannah prayed.

Hannah went with her husband to the holy place of worship. She offered a silent prayer.

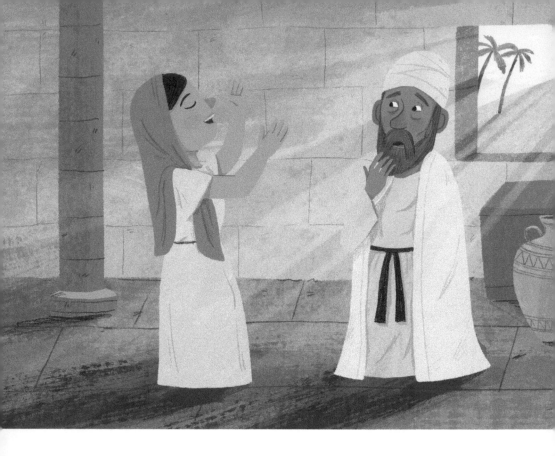

She sent it to God from deep inside her heart. Her
lips moved. But she didn't make a sound. Only God
heard her prayer. Eli the priest was watching. He
thought Hannah was acting silly! Hannah told Eli
she was praying. She was talking to God about her
sadness. It was a sadness only He could understand.
Eli told her, "Go in peace. May God give you what you
ask of Him."

Hannah went home. She felt more hopeful than
ever! Before long, she was pregnant. Her first son

was Samuel. He spent his life serving God. God turned Hannah's never-ending hope into five more children for her to love.

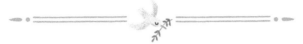

Hannah said: "The Lord has filled my heart with joy. I feel very strong in the Lord. I am glad because You have helped me! There is no one holy like the Lord. There is no God but You. There is no Rock like our God."

1 Samuel 2:1–2

Just like with Hannah, God hears every word you pray. Does Hannah's story help you feel hopeful? Why? Ask God to help you move from simple hope to full-on faith!

THE SHEPHERD
WHO SLAYED
A GIANT

1 SAMUEL 16–17

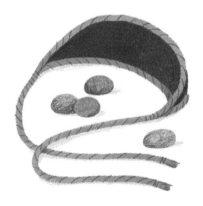

David was a shepherd, living in Israel.
When he was a young man, the
Israelites were in a standoff with
the Philistines. It was getting *messy*.
Every day, the giant Goliath came out of the

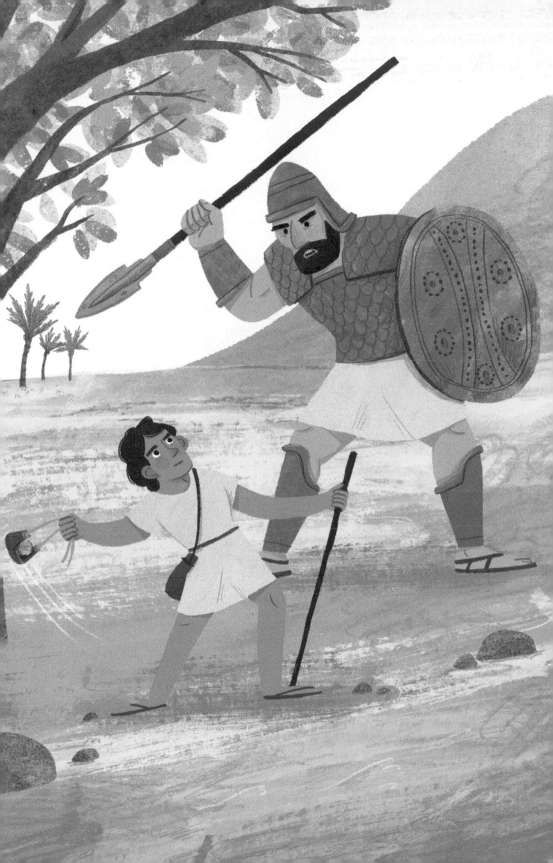

Philistine camp. He was over nine feet tall! He challenged the army of Israel.

Goliath shouted, "Today I stand and dare the army of Israel! Send one of your men to fight me!" He did this for forty days. He shouted it every morning and every evening. King Saul and his army heard the giant's words. They were afraid. They'd forgotten all the miraculous things God had done for them in the past. Their courage shrank to the size of a pea. But God had a plan only He could see.

David said to the king, "Don't be discouraged. I will fight this Philistine!" No one thought this young shepherd had a chance against the giant. But David had the *heart* of a giant. That was all God needed to defend His people.

The giant made fun of David. But David reminded Goliath, "You come at me with a sword. I come to you in the name of the Lord!" David took a stone from his pouch. He put it into his sling and slung it. The stone hit Goliath in the forehead. Down the giant went! Israel expected a warrior to save them. God sent a shepherd instead.

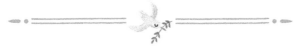

The Lord said to Samuel, "God does not
see the same way people see. People look
at the outside of a person, but the Lord
looks at the heart."

1 Samuel 16:7

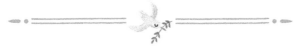 *What helps you feel confident when you're confronted with a challenge? Do you give yourself a pep talk? Do you pray? Think of times when you've had to take a stand for yourself.*

SOLOMON'S PLEASING PRAYER

1 KINGS 3

David grew up to be a king of Israel. God showed kindness and love to King David. The king's tenth son, Solomon, learned to serve God. Solomon served with a faithful heart. He became king at twelve years old after his father died! Solomon soon proved to God he was wise. He had the wisdom of a person who had lived much longer.

God appeared to Solomon in a dream. He told Solomon to ask for whatever he wanted. Young Solomon didn't want wealth. He didn't pray for praise or attention. He didn't ask for

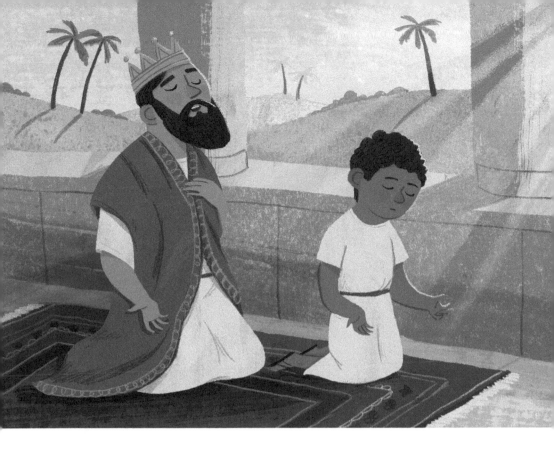

any sort of fancy thing. In his prayer, Solomon first gave gratitude to God. He thanked God for being kind to his father. Then Solomon said, "I'm only a little child. I don't know how to do all the duties of a king!"

Solomon could have had anything in the whole wide world. But he asked God to help him be a good and fair king! Solomon wasn't selfish. He asked God for a wise heart to serve *others*.

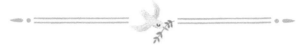

The Lord was pleased that Solomon had asked Him for this. So God said to him, "I will give you wisdom and understanding. Your wisdom will be greater than anyone has had in the past. And there will never be anyone in the future like you."

1 Kings 3:10–12

❓ *When you pray, it's perfectly okay to ask God to take care of you and your needs. But do you also ask God to guide you in helping others? It makes your heart happy when you do something nice for someone.*

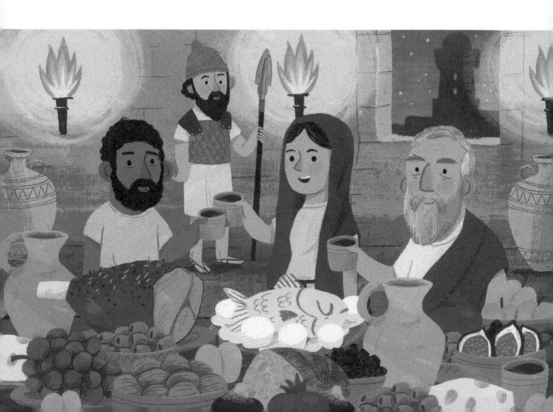

THE ONE TRUE GOD LIGHTS ONE BIG FIRE!

1 KINGS 18

Elijah was a **prophet** for the Lord. Ahab was king of Israel at the time. King Ahab was disobeying God. Ahab ignored God's love. He built an altar for an **idol** known as Baal. God warned His people not to put other gods before Him. Ahab did it anyway!

But God had an idea. He would prove Baal was a false idol. God told Elijah to meet with Ahab. Elijah told Ahab to invite people to come to Mount Carmel. Ahab invited people from all over Israel. This included 450 prophets of Baal.

Elijah told them to prepare a wooden altar for sacrifice. "Ask your god, Baal, to set fire to the altar!" said Elijah. The prophets called on Baal. They prayed and danced. But not a single spark happened. Elijah built an altar. He built his altar in the name of the Lord. He asked for water to be poured onto the wood *three* times. Now it was soaking wet and harder to light!

Elijah prayed, "Oh, Lord, answer me. Show everyone You are the one true God. Show that You love them faithfully and forever." Fire fell. It burned up the wood! It dried the puddles of water! The people praised God. They turned their hearts back to His never-ending love.

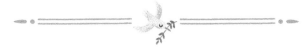

Elijah went near the altar. He prayed, "Lord, answer my prayer. Show these people that You, Lord, are God. Then the people will know that You are bringing them back to You."

1 Kings 18:36–37

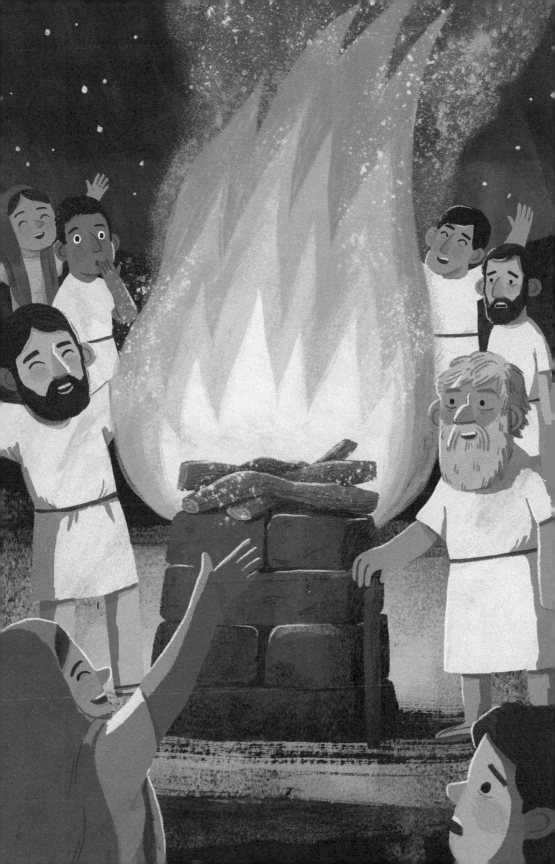

? *What do you see in the world around you that makes you say, "Wow! Look what God can do"? The world often comes with huge challenges, which usually lead to positive change. God's* **miracles** *are real!*

A PRAYER FOR WISDOM AND HOPE

Dear God,

Give me a wise heart. Give me strong hope that has *no* doubt in You! You see everything I'm going through. And every word You say is true.

A BEAUTIFUL QUEEN WITH A BOLD HEART

BOOK OF ESTHER

King Xerxes was a powerful king of Persia. He ruled over 127 countries! The king searched for a wife. He fell in love with a girl who was Jewish. By this time, the Israelites had become known as Jewish people, or Jews. The girl's name was Esther. She became his queen. She was bright and beautiful. The king soon discovered she was brave, too.

Esther's uncle, Mordecai, told her to keep it secret that she was Jewish because he heard

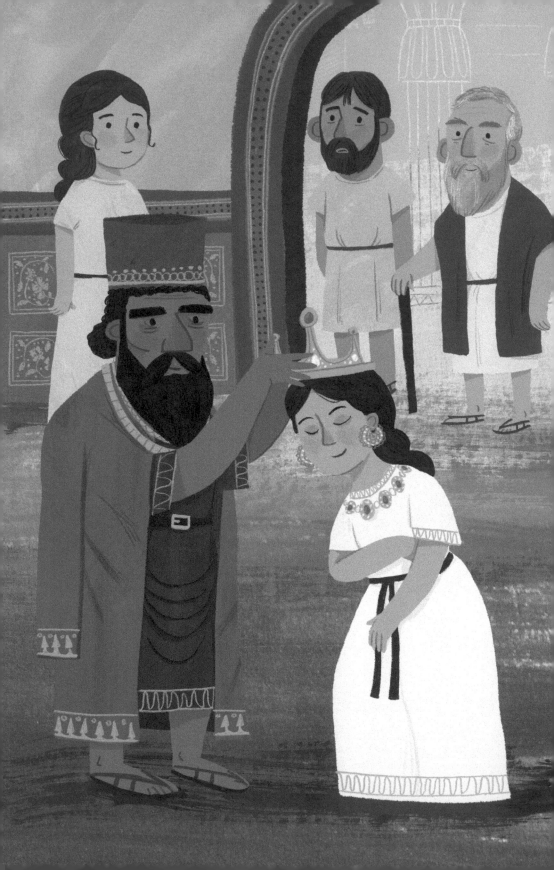

that a bad man named Haman worked for King Xerxes. Haman didn't like Jewish people. He ordered that they be destroyed. Mordecai made sure Esther knew about Haman's plot. Esther was wise and brave. She knew how to save her people and her own life, too. God showed Esther how to carry out His plan at the perfect time, in the perfect way.

Esther went to see King Xerxes. She went without an invitation. It was against the law to go uninvited. Esther was risking death for break-ing the law. She told the king of Haman's hateful 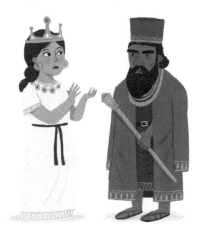 plan. The king listened to Esther. He wrote letters to the countries in the kingdom. He told them to ignore Haman's horrible **mandate**. God's great love moved through Esther's courage. She followed God's plan. *Many* lives were saved!

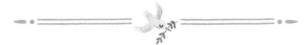

Mordecai gave orders to say to Esther:
"Who knows, you may have been chosen
queen for just such a time as this."

Esther 4:13–14

? *God's plan is sometimes **much** bigger than anyone can imagine. Is there someone you are afraid to approach about something—maybe a teacher or parent? Ask God for courage, and then place your trust in Him like Esther did.*

A PROPHET PREDICTS THE COMING SAVIOR

ISAIAH 9

saiah was a prophet. He had a special assignment from God. Isaiah announced to the world that a king was coming. Isaiah told everyone about the birth of Jesus! Jesus was the most *important* king of all. Jesus was coming to earth to heal the world. He would build a bridge to Heaven, our forever home. Adam and Eve's sin had broken the bridge. In the whole universe, only Jesus could repair it. Jesus is God's only son. His perfect heart is the *only* thing that could save us!

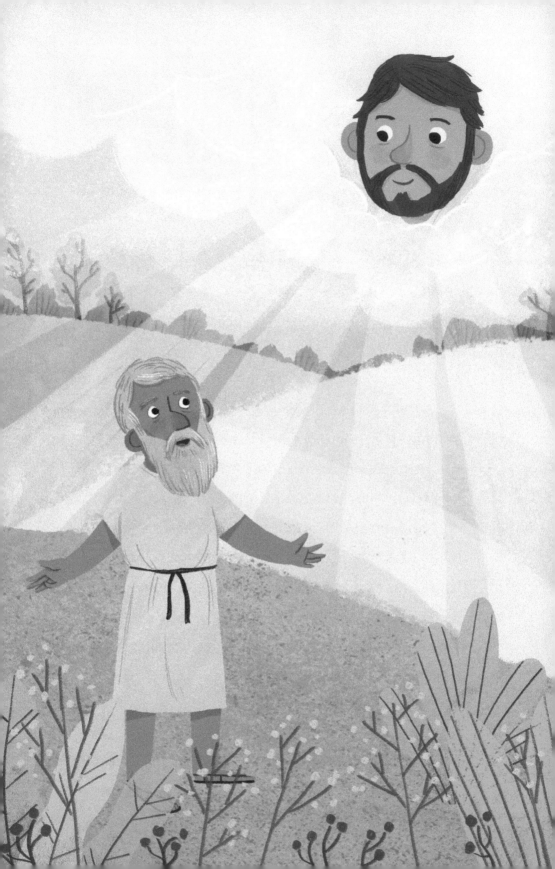

God promised everything would be brighter. He promised everyone would feel lighter. Isaiah described Jesus as a Great Light, Wonderful **Counselor**, Mighty God, Everlasting Father, and Prince of Peace. Isaiah told the world that Jesus is the Savior and King.

Isaiah said that this King wouldn't live in a big castle. He wouldn't wear fancy robes. He did not plan to wear a jeweled crown. The only wealth he brought to earth is the **eternal** love of God. His life would show that God's love is what our hearts need most of all!

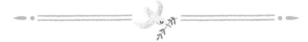

A child will be born to us. God will give a son to us. He will be responsible for leading the people. Power and peace will be in His kingdom.

Isaiah 9:6–7

❓ *Do you know you're the reason Jesus was born? It's true. The truest hope of God's heart is that **every** person learns to love and trust Jesus so that they can live with Him forever. Who are some people in your life who show you God's forever love?*

THREE VERY COOL MEN

DANIEL 3

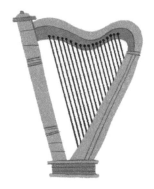

Shadrach, Meshach, and Abednego were brave Israelites. They were officers during the **reign** of proud King Nebuchadnezzar, the Babylonian king. This king had a big gold statue built of himself. He commanded all people to bow down to it. They were to bow whenever they heard the sound of a musical instrument.

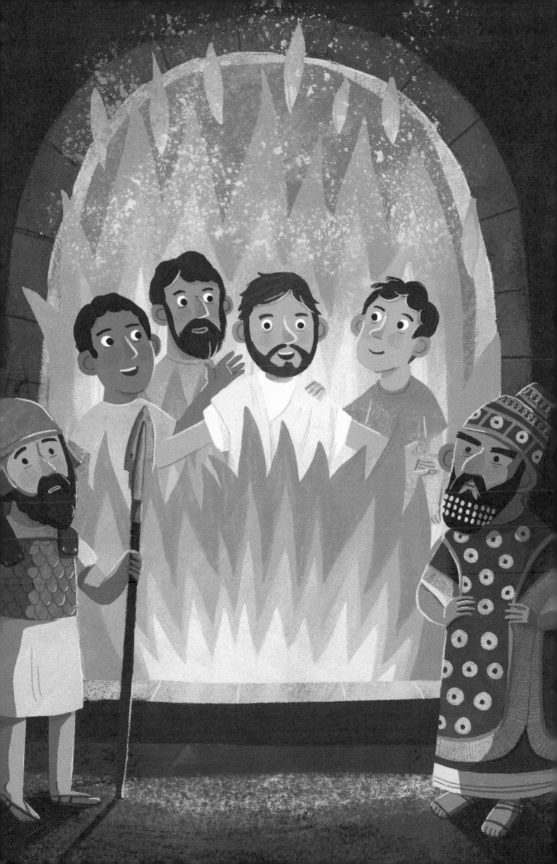

They bowed when they heard horns. They bowed when they heard flutes. They bowed at the sounds of **zithers**, harps, and pipes. What a noisy command!

Shadrach, Meshach, and Abednego refused. They would not bow down to the gold statue. They would not bow now. They would not bow ever. God had told the Israelites to worship only Him. They knew God loved them. And they loved Him back. Their faith in His promises would *never* slack. King Nebuchadnezzar heard about this. The king was mad. He called for the three men. They told the king, "We will not serve your gods. We will not worship the statue you built."

"*Grrrrr*," the king huffed. "My furnace isn't quite *hot* enough. Heat it seven times hotter. Then tie up these men and throw them in!" But soon the king noticed one more. *Four* men were in the furnace. And not one was burned. God sent an angel to protect the three men. They had obeyed His commandment. King Nebuchadnezzar's heart was changed by what he saw. He learned that God's love is the mightiest of all!

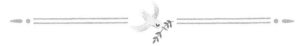

Nebuchadnezzar said, "Praise the God of Shadrach, Meshach and Abednego. Their God has sent His angel and saved His servants from the fire!"

Daniel 3:28

? *Doing what pleases God can be hard, but it's always right! What helps you stay brave when you choose to do the right thing? God will always send courage when you trust in Him!*

DANIEL SLUMBERS WITH THE LIONS

King Darius, the Babylonian King, loved Daniel, who was a prophet. He supervised a large group of **governors**. Daniel was an honest, loyal leader. The king planned to put Daniel in charge of the whole kingdom. Other supervisors and governors became jealous. They decided to make Daniel look bad.

Daniel loved God. He prayed every day. The scheming governors convinced the king to make a new law. The law stated no one could

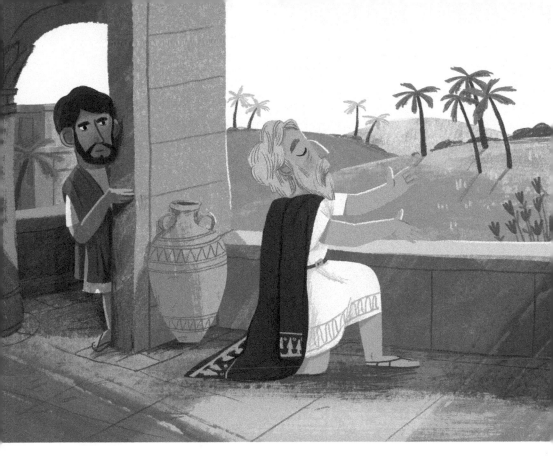

worship anyone but King Darius for thirty days. They saw Daniel praying to God. They went straight to the king to tattle! King Darius was sad that Daniel broke the law. The king knew Daniel would be thrown into the lions' den.

The den was sealed with a stone after Daniel was tossed in. King Darius spent the whole night worrying. He secretly hoped Daniel's God would save him. At sunrise the king ran to the den. He removed the stone. He yelled, "Daniel! Was your God able to save you?"

"Yes!" Daniel shouted. "My God sent His angel to close the lions' mouths." Daniel's night in the lions' den was more like a slumber party!

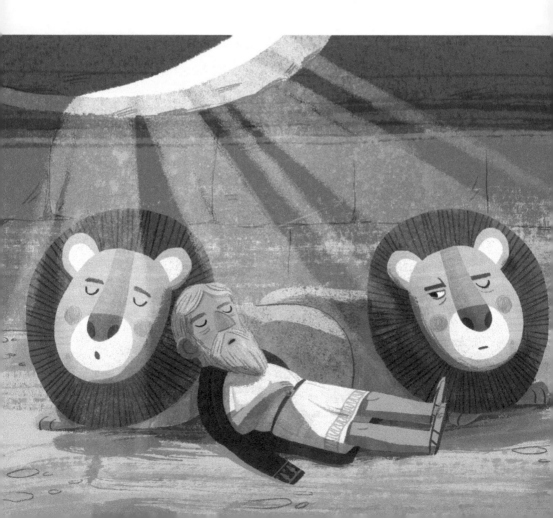

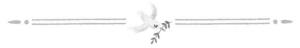

Then King Darius wrote a letter. It was to all people and all nations, to those who spoke every language in the world: All of you must respect the God of Daniel. Daniel's God is the living God. His rule will never end. God does mighty miracles. God saved Daniel from the power of the lions.

Daniel 6:25–27

Daniel showed more than bravery in the lions' den—he firmly demonstrated faith. Daniel's safety came from his faith in God. When do you feel most protected by God's love? Practice staying in faith!

ONE BIG GULP

JONAH 1–3

Jonah loved God. Usually, he listened to God. He was happy to obey. But then God told Jonah to go to Nineveh to preach. Jonah crossed his arms. He turned his back. He marched to the dock. He bought a ticket to sail to a different city!

Soon into its **voyage**, the ship was caught in a terrible storm. The captain shook Jonah from his nap. He said, "Wake up! Pray to your god so he might save us!" Jonah knew the trouble they were in was his doing. It was God's way of getting his attention. Jonah knew how to save the ship.

"Throw me into the sea," Jonah said. "I serve the Lord of heaven. He made the sea and the land.

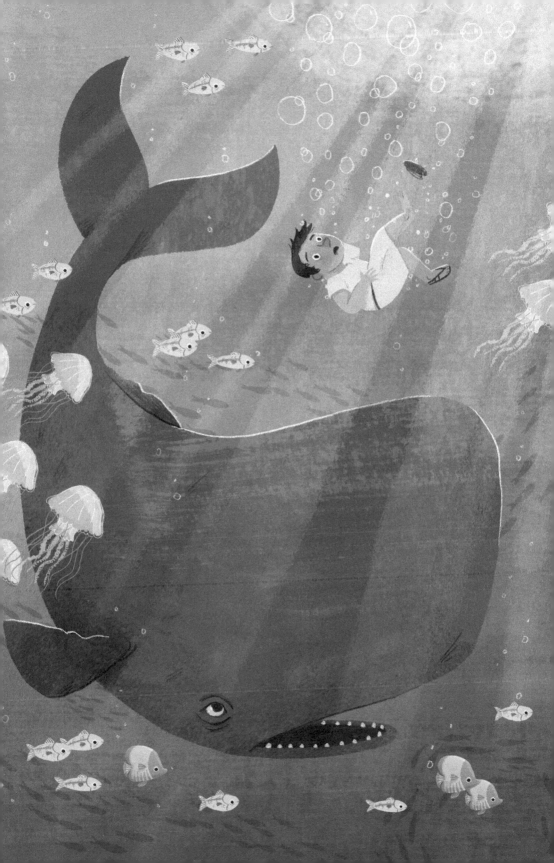

This great wind is my fault. I turned away from God."
The crew tossed Jonah overboard. The sea went calm.

Jonah was sinking. Down, down, down he sank.
His hope, too, sank. But God loved Jonah. He sent a big
fish. The fish swallowed Jonah in one big gulp! Jonah
spent three days and nights in the stinky, sloppy belly
of the fish. Jonah prayed. He promised **loyalty** to God.

The fish let out a belch. *Burp!* It spit Jonah onto
dry land. God spoke to Jonah again. This time, Jonah
went straight to Nineveh! Jonah listened to God. The
people listened to Jonah. And that's how God's love
saved Nineveh!

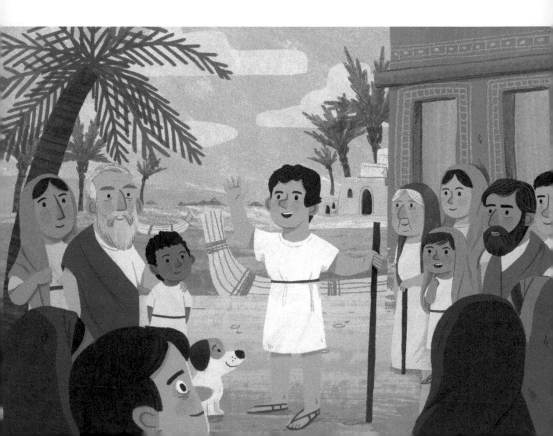

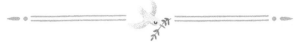

While Jonah was in the stomach of the fish, he prayed to the Lord his God. Jonah said, "You threw me into the sea. Your powerful waves flowed over me. Seaweed wrapped around my head. But You saved me from death. Salvation comes from the Lord!"

Jonah 2:1–9

? *Jonah told the people of Nineveh to stop doing wrong and start serving God—because God's love had **never** left them. Do you feel there's an issue in your life you should steer in another direction? Like Jonah, take some time to think about better choices you might make.*

A PRAYER FOR A LISTENING HEART

Dear God,

Help me listen to You with all my heart and remember the good things You say. Goodness and peace are what You give when I follow Your words every day.

THE NEW TESTAMENT

FROM HEAVEN TO EARTH— JESUS IS HERE!

LUKE 1–2

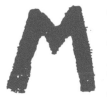ary was a young Jewish girl from Nazareth. She was engaged to a young man named Joseph. Before their wedding day arrived, Mary got a surprise visit. God sent an angel. The angel, Gabriel, had a message. "God has blessed you," he told Mary. At first, she wasn't sure what he meant. She felt blessed by God's love every day!

Gabriel told Mary she would become pregnant. She would give birth to a son. His name

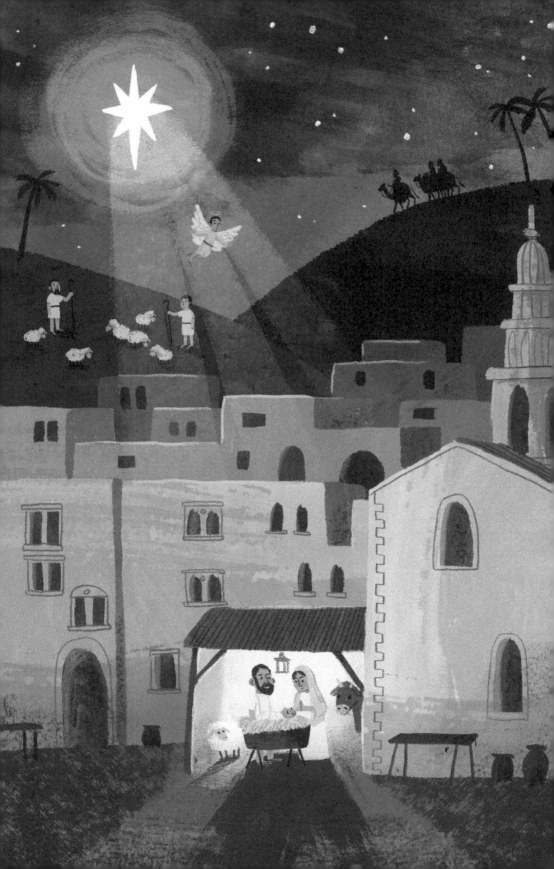

would be Jesus. He would save the people from sin. Mary felt happy. God had chosen her for something very special. "I am the Lord's servant. Let this happen to me as you say," she told Gabriel.

Many months later, Joseph and Mary traveled to the town of Bethlehem. When they arrived, the city was overcrowded. There was nowhere for them to sleep. Mary was ready to have her baby. They had to stay in a stable, where animals were kept. Joseph made her as comfortable as he could. It was a warm shelter. It was a **humble** beginning for a baby who would become King. King Jesus was finally here to show us the way!

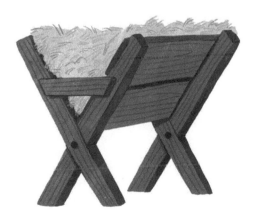

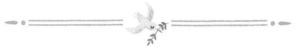

Shepherds were in the fields nearby watching their sheep. An angel of the Lord said to them, "Today your Savior was born in David's town. He is Christ, the Lord. This is how you will know Him: You will find a baby wrapped in cloths and lying in a feeding box."

Luke 2:8–12

? *How is Jesus different from other kings you've read about in Bible stories? What do you think is the most important quality in a king? What do you love most about Jesus?*

JESUS PRAYS FOR THE CHILDREN

MATTHEW 19

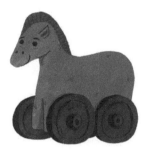

As Jesus grew, He began to teach. He taught about God and called a special group to teach with him. They were called **disciples**. Jesus and his disciples were busy. They were going about the land. They healed the sick. They loved others. They taught how to live the way of God. *Whew!* Sometimes they got tired. They needed a rest.

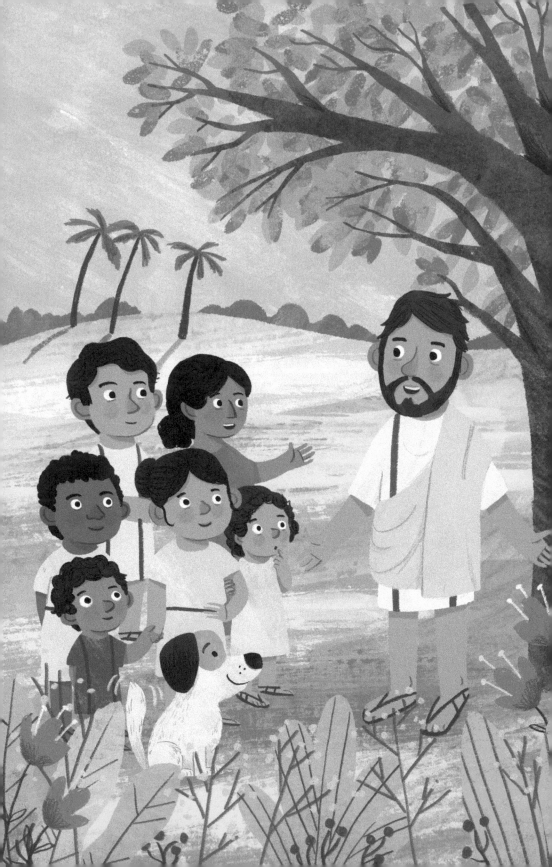

One busy day, a group of parents brought their children to Jesus. They wanted Him to pray for them. Jesus was happy. He scooped the children into His arms! But Jesus's followers thought He might want to spend time doing something else. They told the parents to stop bringing the children. Those followers were wrong!

Jesus told His followers to *never* stop the children from visiting with Him. The children's hearts were pure—like those God welcomed into his kingdom of heaven! Jesus taught everyone something good that day. Children have an incredibly special place in God's heart. God's love for little children is as big as the universe and beyond!

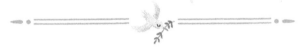

Jesus said, "Let the little children come to me. Don't stop them, because the kingdom of heaven belongs to people who are like these children."

Matthew 19:14

? *Do you know that Jesus prays for **you**? What do you share with Him when you pray? You can tell Him **anything**, and He will **always** love you.*

JESUS STILLS STORMY WATERS

MARK 4

One day Jesus was near a lake. He was teaching a crowd of people. He told **parables** to help them understand God's love. These stories inspired people to live for God. Jesus hopped into a boat along the shore. That way, everyone could see and hear Him. In the evening, He finished teaching. He told the disciples to jump into the boat. They would cross the lake together.

Jesus went to the back of the boat. He put His head down and fell right to sleep. Maybe that's why He didn't hear the wind. It started

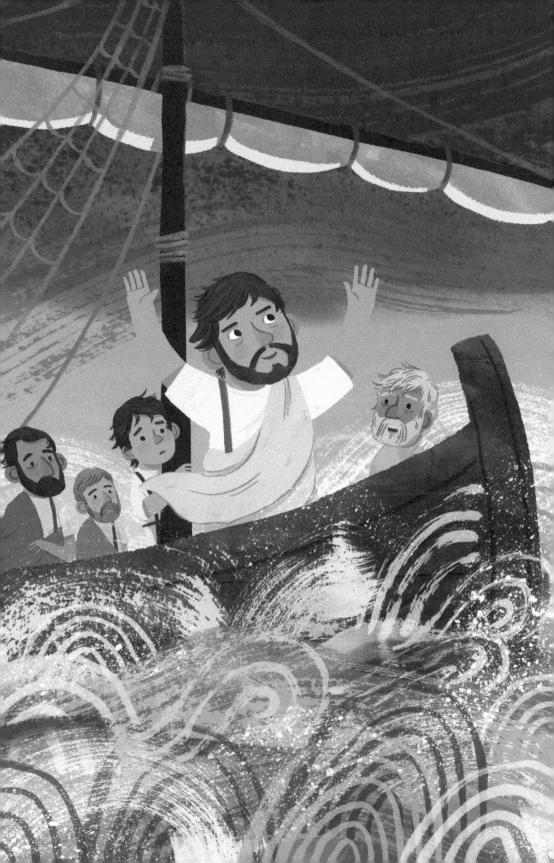

to howl. The waves began to swell. Water in the boat was rising. So was fear in the minds of the disciples!

They worried about the storm crashing around them. They decided to wake their Master. Jesus stood up. He shouted three words: "Quiet! Be still." The wind stopped. The waves calmed. The disciples were thankful they weren't going to drown! Jesus asked, "Why are you afraid? Do you still doubt God's care for you?"

The disciples looked at one another with wide, surprised eyes. "Even the wind and the waves obey Him," they said. After seeing this miracle, their faith in Jesus grew stronger.

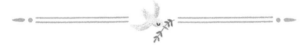

The followers were very afraid and asked each other, "What kind of man is this? Even the wind and the waves obey Him!"

Mark 4:41

❓ *Do you ever let doubt creep in, causing you to question your faith in God? Think of ways you might change your thinking to shed doubt and regain trust in God. He can help you clear **any** hurdle.*

A LIFE OF LOVE AND BLESSING

MATTHEW 5

Jesus was in the city of Galilee. He saw a large crowd gathering. He made His way to a hilltop. He sat down to teach them how to live a blessed life. Word was spreading throughout the land. Jesus was helping people learn God's ways. They loved His simple stories and instructions. The people sat on the hillside. Jesus taught eight truths of a blessed life:

1. Those who rely on God are blessed. Heaven is their forever home.

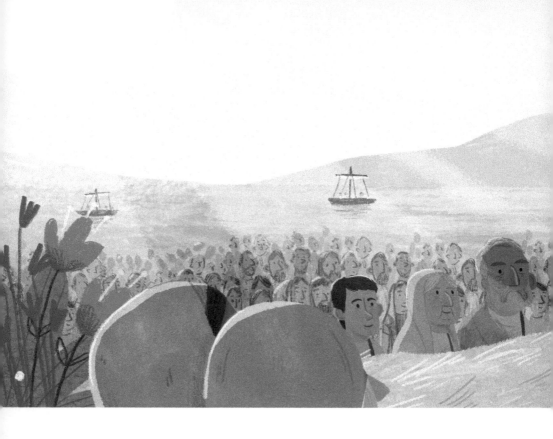

2. Those who are sad now will be loved. God will **comfort** them.

3. Those who are humble are blessed. They'll enjoy good things on earth.

4. Those who always want to do what's right are blessed. God will fully provide for them.

5. Those who forgive are blessed. **Forgiveness** will be given to them in return.

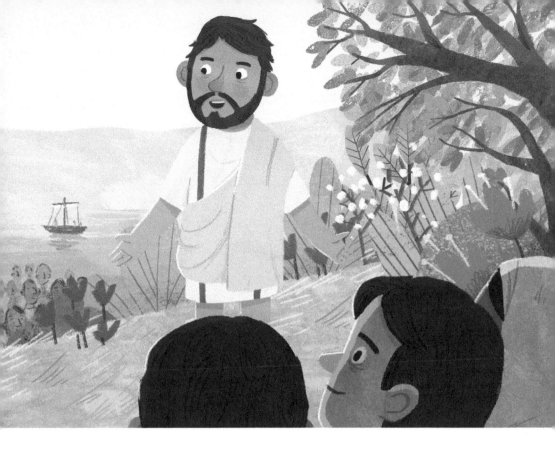

6. Those who are positive in thought are blessed. They are in the presence of God.

7. Those who live in peace are blessed. God will call them His children.

8. Those who do good are blessed, even if they are treated badly for it. The kingdom of heaven belongs to them.

Jesus taught the people that even when hard things happen to us, or we get sad, or someone picks on us for doing good and listening to Him, God's love and blessings are available to everyone.

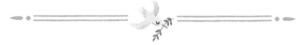

People will say bad things about you and hurt you. They will lie and say all kinds of evil things about you because you follow Me. But when they do these things to you, you are happy. Rejoice and be glad. You have a great reward waiting for you in heaven.

Matthew 5:11–12

When you have felt sad, who or what has God put in your life to cheer you up?

THE GOOD NEIGHBOR

LUKE 10

A teacher of God's law spoke to Jesus. The teacher said, "The law says we must love God with all our heart, strength, and soul. We are also told to love our neighbor. Who is the neighbor?" To answer the question Jesus told a parable.

"A man was walking," Jesus said. "A group of robbers attacked him. They took all his belongings. They left him lying by the road. A **religious** leader saw the hurt man. He crossed the road without doing a thing! Another man came along. He stopped to look at the suffering man. But he, too, decided not to help."

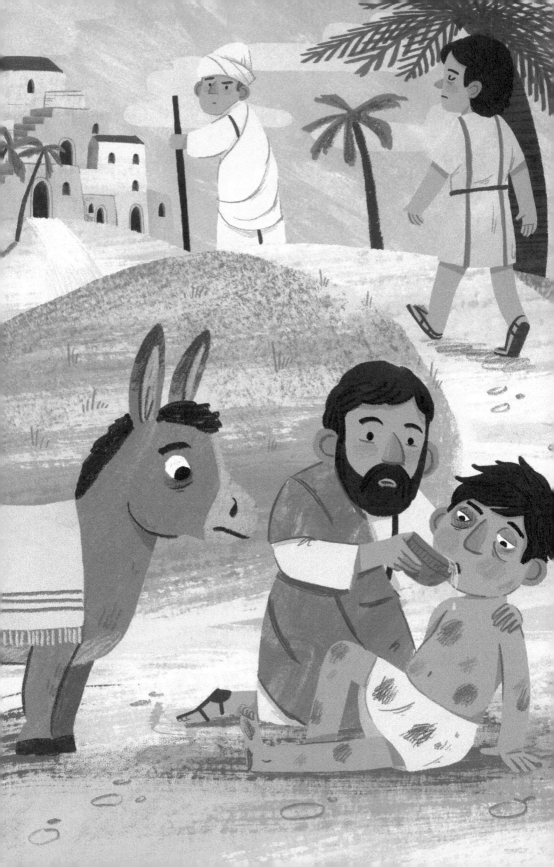

Jesus continued, "Then a man from Samaria saw the injured man. He felt sad for him. He knelt down. He bandaged the man's wounds. He lifted the man onto his donkey. The good Samaritan took him to an inn. He told the innkeeper, 'Let the injured man stay until he is well enough to leave. I'll return to pay whatever it costs.'"

Jesus then told the teacher he should do as the good Samaritan did! A person in need is our neighbor, no matter where they come from. God's love in us should always act kindly and show compassion toward others.

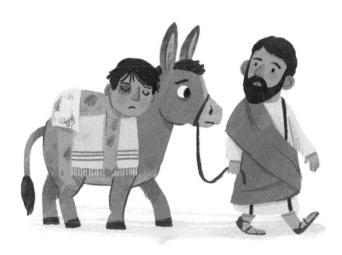

Jesus said, "Which one of these three men do you think was a neighbor to the man who was attacked by the robbers?" The teacher of the law answered, "The one who helped him."

Luke 10:36–37

Have you had the chance to help someone in need? If so, who? If not, can you think of ways you could help others? Maybe you could donate the clothes you've outgrown, or perhaps an elderly neighbor needs someone to weed her garden.

A SON WHO MADE A SILLY DECISION

LUKE 15

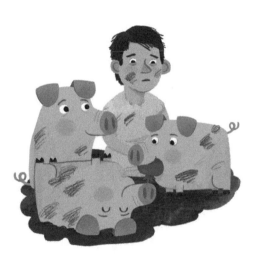

Jesus once told a story about a man with two sons. The younger son decided life at his father's house was boring. So he traveled far from home. He took with him his share of the family money. He spent the money on foolish things.

Before long, his money ran out. He was without money or food. The boy was sad and hungry. He went to a local farmer. He got a job on the farm. But the farmer did not pay him fairly. The boy was so hungry even the husks he fed the pigs looked yummy. *Yuck!*

I have to go home, the boy thought. *I'll tell my father I'm sorry. Maybe he'll forgive me.* He was sure his father would be angry, but the boy went home.

His father ran to him when he arrived. He gave his son a big hug. "Welcome home, son!"

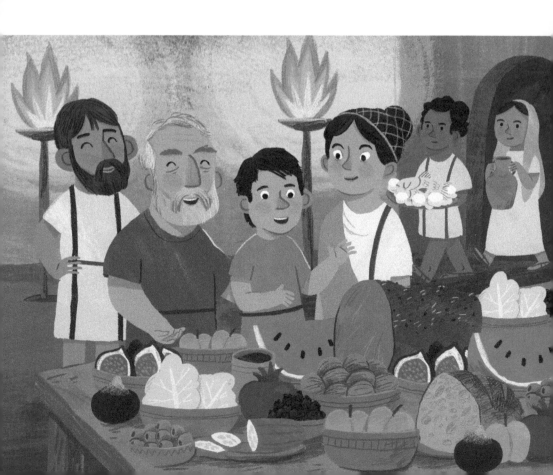

The boy said, "I'm sorry, father. I made a silly decision. It made you *and* God unhappy."

The father forgave his son. He told his servants to prepare a feast. "My son was in the wrong place. Now he's in the right place: back in my loving arms!"

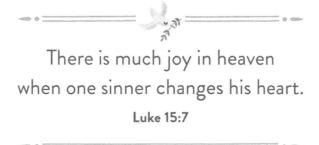

There is much joy in heaven
when one sinner changes his heart.

Luke 15:7

❓ *Do you feel comfortable talking to God when you've made a mistake? He will always be there with open arms!*

A PRAYER TO STAY HUMBLE WHEN WE STUMBLE!

Dear God,

When I make a mistake or turn away, You welcome me back with arms open wide! You're a perfect Father in every way, and I *never* have to hide.

A MIRACLE FROM A LITTLE BOY'S LUNCH

JOHN 6

It had been a long day of teaching. Jesus crossed a lake for some quiet time. He rested on a grassy field. He saw thousands of people coming toward him. They'd seen him do many miracles. They were excited to hear more of his teachings.

It was near dinnertime. They needed to feed the crowd. Jesus asked a disciple where they could buy bread. "A person would have to work a long, long time to buy bread for all these people!" the disciple told Jesus.

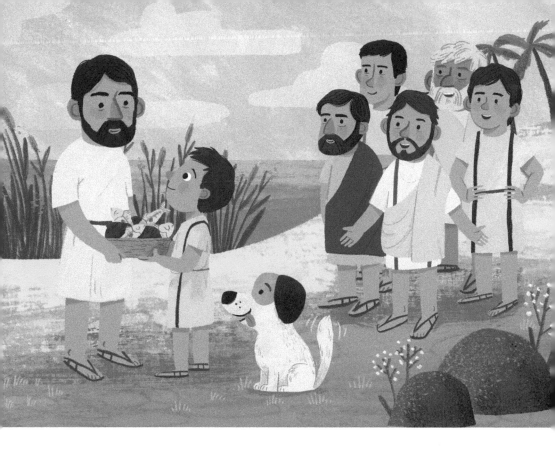

Another disciple tried to help. A boy offered his lunch of five loaves of bread and two little fish. It wasn't nearly enough to feed the crowd. Jesus knew God had a plan.

Jesus thanked God for the food. He told the disciples to pass around the bread and fish. They passed the food basket. It filled up with more fish and bread! All 5,000 people ate. Their bellies were full! God even provided leftovers. They could feed *more* people if they came to listen to Jesus.

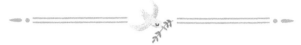

They all had enough to eat. When they had finished, Jesus said to his followers, "Gather the pieces of fish and bread that were not eaten. Don't waste anything."

John 6:12–13

? *Jesus knows God **always** provides what we need. God's love for us is **big**. He loves to give and give! Is there something you'd like to thank God for today?*

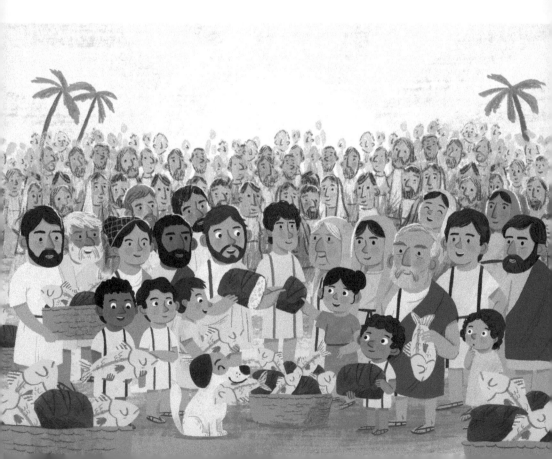

JESUS
STEPS OUT . . .
ON WATER!

MARK 6

Jesus told His disciples to row in a boat across the lake. He would meet them later. He wanted time alone to pray. Jesus understood the importance of talking with God. He knew it made Him strong!

Jesus finished praying. He went to the lake. He saw His disciples rowing. They rowed with all their might. But wind blew against the boat. They couldn't move in the direction they wanted to go. Jesus quickly walked out on the

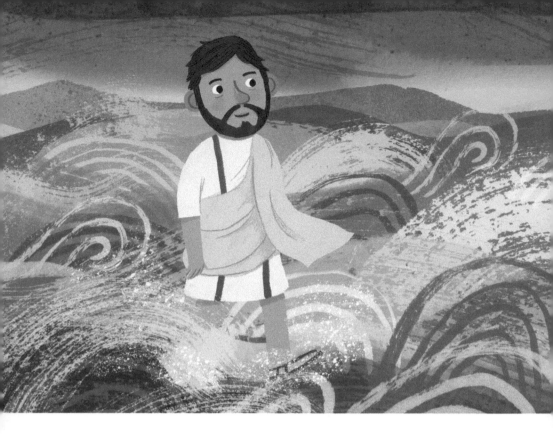

water to help! He walked as if the water were as solid as the ground.

The disciples saw His figure walking toward them. They did not recognize Him. It was dark. Water splashed in their eyes. They were tired. "It's a ghost!" they cried. They were afraid.

Jesus told them, "Be brave! It is I! You have *nothing* to fear." The disciples heard Jesus's voice. They calmed down. He stepped into the boat. The water, too, calmed down. Jesus was now by their side. It was smooth sailing straight to the shore.

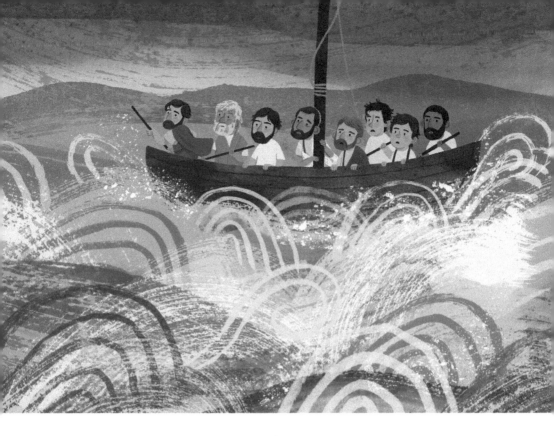

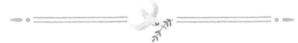

When they had crossed the lake, they came
to the shore at Gennesaret. They tied the
boat there. People saw Jesus and immedi-
ately recognized Him. They ran to tell others
everywhere in that area that Jesus was there.

Mark 6:53–55

❓ *When something seems impossible, remember that anything
is possible with God! Have you ever had a challenge that seems
too hard for you to meet? God will lift you up!*

TWO SISTERS
AND A TANTRUM

LUKE 10

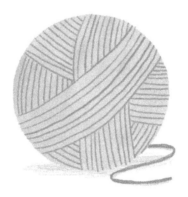

A woman named Martha welcomed Jesus into her home. Martha loved to be a good hostess. Guests often stayed with her. She spun yarn. She mended clothing. She cooked and baked. It didn't matter how much time it would take!

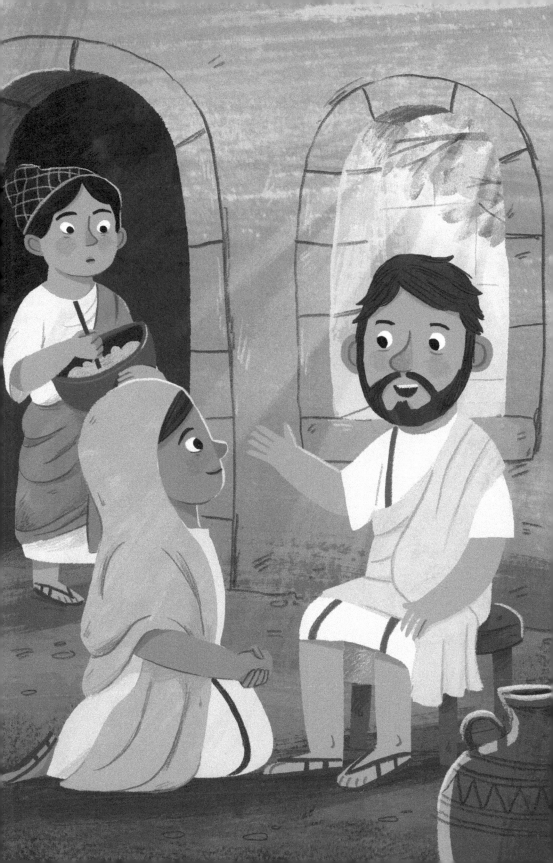

Martha had a sister named Mary. Jesus sat down to teach. Mary sat down to listen. She was listening carefully. She was learning happily. She was hearing about God's love. She smiled joyfully! Mary paid close attention to Jesus. Meanwhile, Martha was busy. She was cleaning up. She was tidying. She was also getting *angry*.

Martha stomped into the room. She said, "Lord, do You see my sister leaving all the work to me? Please tell her to help!"

Jesus answered, "Martha, you're worried about so many little things. You've forgotten about what is most important! Why are you upset? Mary is growing in God's love. It's a gift that can *never* be taken from her."

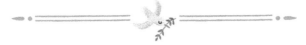

Jesus called the people to Him again. He said, "Every person should listen to Me and understand what I am saying."

Mark 7:14

? *Like Mary, do you enjoy learning about God's love for you? What are some ways you might help others know God's love? You could share a story with friends, or simply show love through kindness.*

A PRAYER TO CHOOSE WHAT'S BEST AND BLESSED

Dear God,

Let me be careful to choose the right things.

Goodness and love are what my choice brings.

JESUS HEALS A LITTLE GIRL

LUKE 8

Jesus was becoming well-known. People were drawn to His teachings. They were in **awe** of His many miracles. The crowds around Him got bigger and bigger! A leader named Jairus met with Jesus. He begged Jesus to come to his house. His only daughter needed help. She was twelve years old. She was dying.

Jesus walked with Jairus to his house. But He was being delayed! People were all around Him. They were trying to touch Him. Jesus was filled with God's love. Everyone wanted to be close to Him.

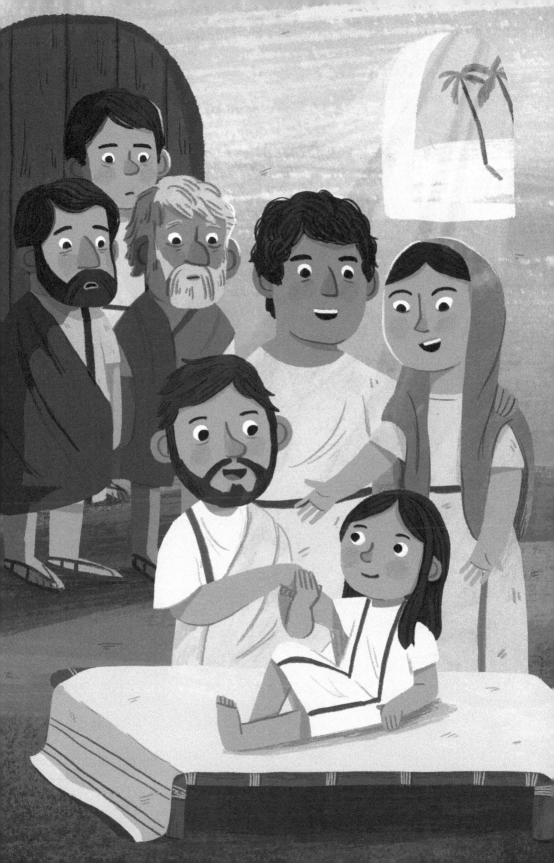

Along the way, they got bad news. Jairus's daughter had died. Jesus told Jairus not to be afraid. He told him to believe his daughter would be okay! Jesus went into the house. Many people were crying. They thought the young girl was dead. Jesus said, "Don't cry. This girl is only sleeping." Some of the people laughed at Him. They didn't believe Jesus. Then Jesus took the little girl's hand. He said, "My child, get up!" Suddenly the girl stood. Her parents were **astonished**!

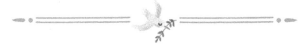

While Jesus was still speaking, someone came from the house of the synagogue ruler and said to the ruler, "Your daughter has died! Don't bother the teacher now." When Jesus heard this, He said to Jairus, "Don't be afraid. Just believe, and your daughter will be well."

Luke 8:49–50

❓ *God's love for us is filled with surprisingly good things! Has something good happened for you or a friend that made you feel especially happy? Did you give God a big thank-You?*

LAZARUS LIVES!

JOHN 11

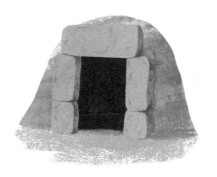

Jesus loved his friend Lazarus. He also loved Lazarus's sisters, Mary and Martha. The sisters sent someone to tell Jesus, "Lazarus is very sick." God was going to send a miracle. Jesus knew it in his heart. Then Lazarus died from his illness. But it was only the beginning of this story.

Jesus arrived in Bethany. Lazarus had been laid in a tomb. Lazarus had been in the tomb for *four* days. Everyone was sad. Lots of friends were there. They tried to comfort

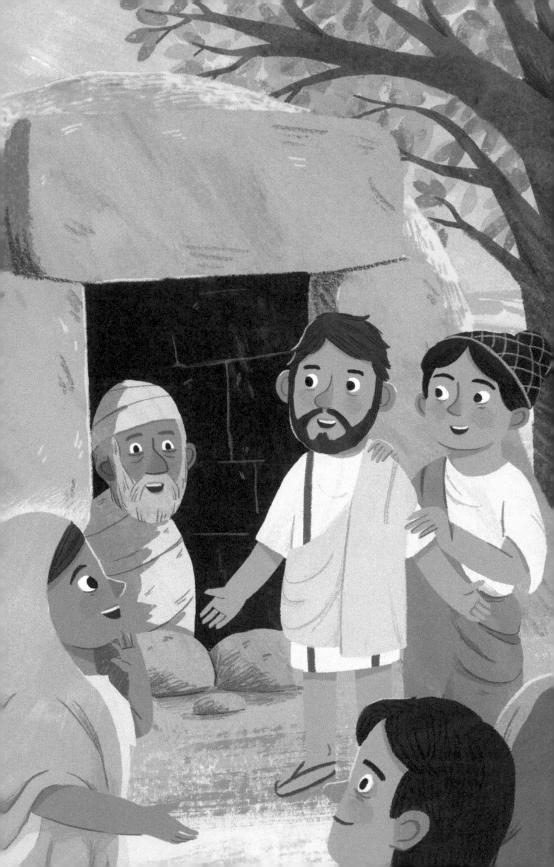

Mary and Martha. They were sure Lazarus's life on earth was over. Jesus cried with his friends.

But Jesus was about to show God's amazing love! First, He thanked God for hearing His prayer. Jesus asked God for a miracle. He knew the miracle would help the people believe. God had sent Jesus to give *everyone* new life—a life that would go on forever. Jesus stood outside the tomb. He said, "Lazarus, come out!" And Lazarus did! Lazarus's new life showed many people why Jesus came to earth. The whole world would have never-ending life with God.

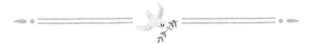

Jesus said, "I am the **resurrection** and the life. He who believes in Me will have life even if he dies. Martha, do you believe this?" Martha answered, "Yes, Lord. I believe that You are the Christ, the Son of God. You are the One Who was coming to the world."

John 11:25–27

How do you overcome sadness? Jesus can help you feel better when you're down. Think about your love for Jesus, and feel comforted.

A SHORT MAN
IN A TALL TREE

LUKE 19

Zacchaeus was a tax collector in the city of Jericho. But he cheated. He collected too much. He kept the extra for himself. Everyone knew about it. Zacchaeus was getting rich! He had no friends or visitors. That is, until Jesus came.

The townspeople heard Jesus was coming. They gathered along the road to see Him. Zacchaeus was short. He stood on tiptoes. He tried to squeeze to the front. He stretched his neck as far as he could. It was no use. He climbed a tall tree to see. He saw Jesus staring up at him! "Come down from there," Jesus said. "I need

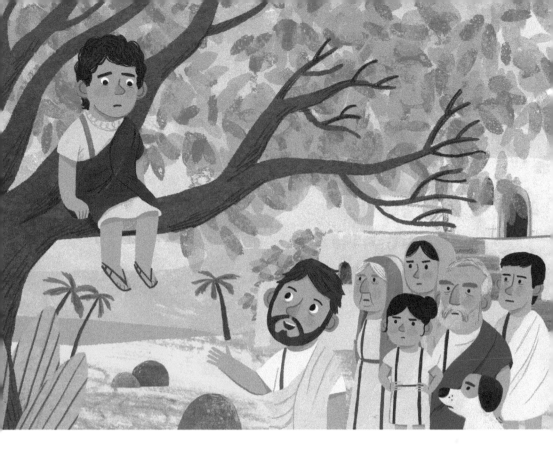

to go to your house today." Zacchaeus felt important!
He also felt his heart sink. He was very sorry for what
he'd done.

Zacchaeus told Jesus, "I'll give back all I've stolen.
Plus, I'll add four times more!" He asked for forgiveness. At first, the people were upset. They didn't like
that Jesus visited Zacchaeus the cheater. But Jesus
taught everyone a lesson that day: God loves us all
the same, no matter what! God's love can change
anyone's heart.

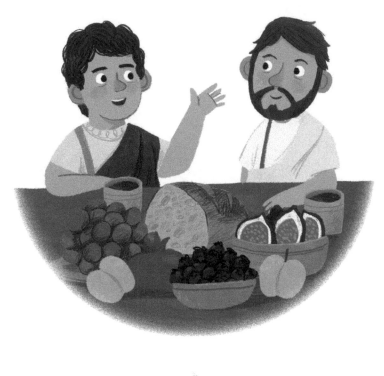

Zacchaeus was pleased to have Jesus in his house.
All the people saw this and began to complain,
"Look at the kind of man Jesus stays with.
Zacchaeus is a sinner!" Jesus said, "Salvation has
come to this house today. The Son of Man came to
find lost people and save them."

Luke 19:6–10

? *God loves everyone the same, no matter what! How does your heart feel when you're sorry for something you've done, and you've apologized? God always forgives. Learn to forgive others. And when you slip up, also forgive yourself.*

A PRAYER THE WORLD WILL SEE GOD'S LOVE IN ME

Dear God,

You forgive me when I make mistakes. You still love me when I do. Give me a heart that's quick to forgive, so I show Your love, too.

JESUS RIDES INTO JERUSALEM

JOHN 12

The time had come for Jesus to enter the city of Jerusalem in Israel. The last part of God's perfect plan, the resurrection, would happen there. Jesus rode in on a donkey. The prophet Zechariah had written it hundreds of years before: *Don't be afraid, people of Jerusalem! Your King is coming. He is sitting on a donkey.*

The people were not afraid. They waved palm branches. They shouted, "Praise God! God bless the One who comes in the name of the Lord! God bless the King of Israel!" They

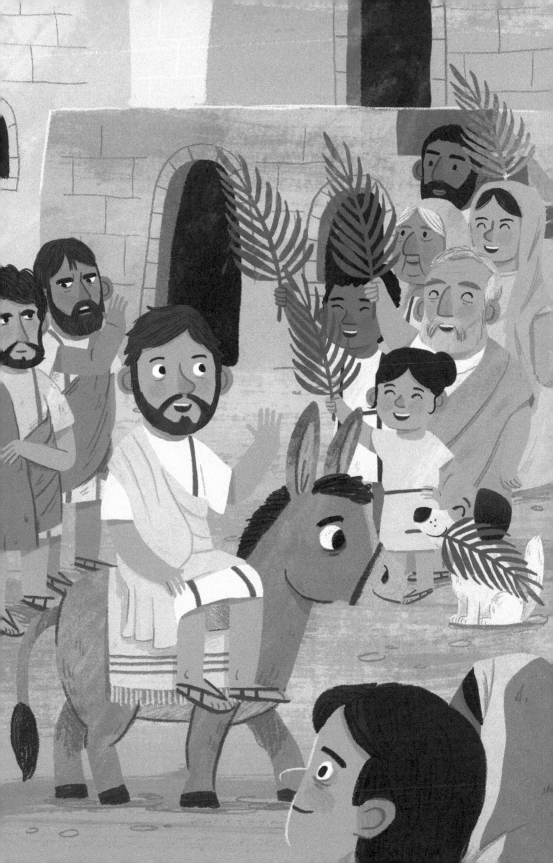

celebrated God's promise. They were happy to see Jesus!

Sadly, the happy welcome didn't last long. Religious leaders wanted to silence Jesus because of the commotion He made. They didn't believe He was the Son of God. They accused Jesus of lying. They would not put their hope in Jesus. They did not like the stories He told. They had stubborn hearts that wouldn't budge. But God's perfect, powerful love would **prevail**! God would prove that *every* word Jesus spoke was true.

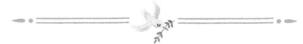

Jesus cried out, "He who believes in Me is really believing in the One Who sent Me. He who sees Me sees the One Who sent Me. I have come as light into the world."

John 12:44–46

? *Has anyone ever made fun of you for believing in Jesus? How do you deal with those moments? God is **always** happy when you go to Him in prayer, so ask Him to help you stay true to Him—despite what others say or think.*

SUPPER
IS SERVED

MARK 14

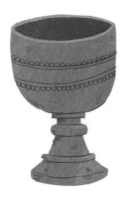

It was the first day of the Passover Feast. It was a time of remembering. God's people remembered being rescued from slavery in Egypt. God wanted them to *always* celebrate this important miracle of His love. Jesus told His disciples to prepare their feast.

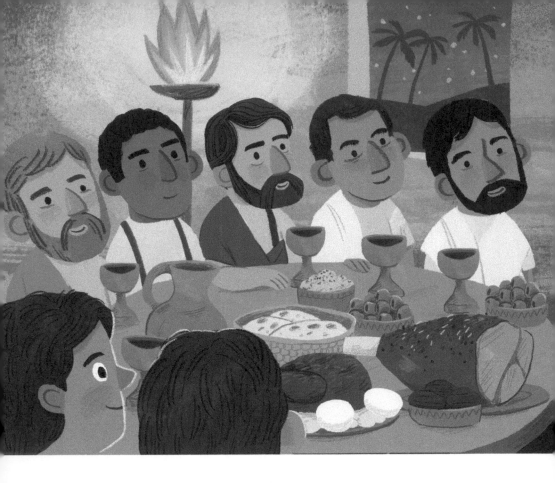

They feasted in the large upstairs room of a house in Jerusalem.

They sat around the table. Jesus said He would soon give His life. This would wash away the sins of the world. God planned to make all hearts pure. He was going to **restore** hope! It was the hope of spending forever with Him. This lasting hope could *never* be smudged again.

Jesus knew this was His last supper. He shared it with the disciples. He thanked God. He broke the

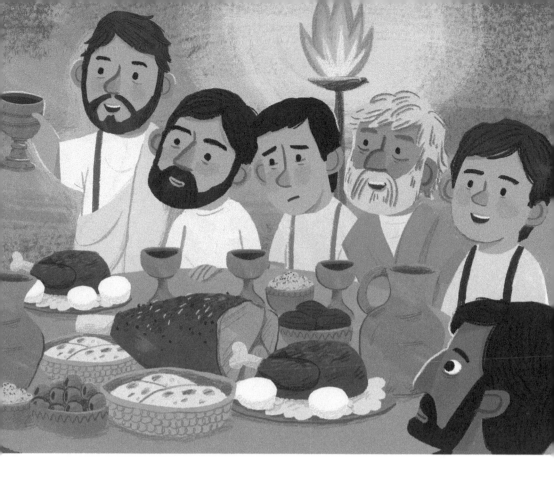

bread into pieces. He said, "My body will be broken like this." Jesus lifted a cup. He drank from it. He passed it around. He said, "My life will be poured out to save the lives of many." They finished their meal. Jesus went to the Mount of Olives. He needed time alone with God. He knew His heart had to be *stronger than ever*. He was going to follow God's perfect plan.

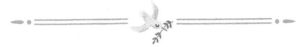

Jesus told the followers, "You will all
lose your faith in Me. It is written in the
Scriptures. But after I rise from death, I will
go ahead of you into Galilee."

Mark 14:27–28

? *When sin came into the world, it put a stain on people's hearts that they couldn't clean off by themselves. God makes us pure. God makes us strong. How often do you ask God for strength? What are some ways He has helped you through a tough time?*

GOOD FRIDAY

MATTHEW 27, LUKE 23

Jesus was done praying. He was in the Garden of Gethsemane. It was time for the world to see what God had planned. His love for all would never be braver or stronger. Jesus, God's only Son, would light the way to heaven. But it would be a painful and lonely path.

Soldiers came into the garden. They carried swords and clubs. Jesus stayed quiet and calm. They arrested Jesus. He went with them willingly. He knew it was part of God's plan. Jesus was taken to religious leaders. They demanded He be killed on a cross. They convinced lots of people to agree with them. Jesus

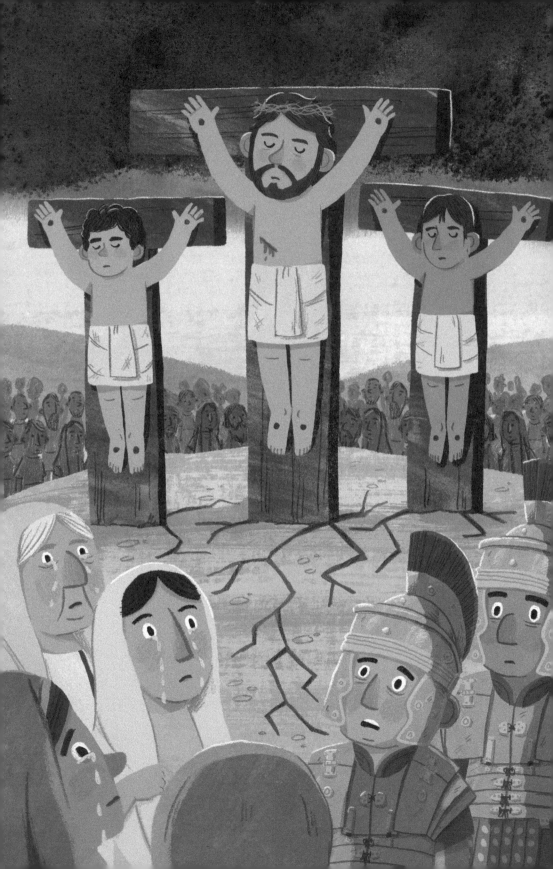

was **innocent**. But the crowd was loud and angry. So the religious leader gave them their way.

Jesus was nailed to a wooden cross. He was left to suffer and die. Those who loved Him cried. Even the sky and the earth felt sad. The sky turned dark for three hours that day. The earth shook. Rocks tumbled. The soldiers saw this. They were scared. They said, *"He really was the son of God!"* And they were right.

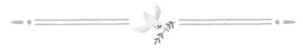

There were also two criminals led out with Jesus. The soldiers nailed the criminals to their crosses beside Jesus. Jesus said, "Father, forgive them. They don't know what they are doing."

Luke 23:32–34

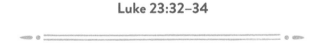

❓ *Sometimes life feels completely unfair. Can you think of a time when you felt you weren't treated fairly? Maybe a friend or sibling blamed you for something you didn't do. What promises from God help you when you want to scream, "Hey, that's not fair!"?*

JESUS IS RISEN!

JOHN 20, MATTHEW 27–28

After Jesus died, His body was laid in a tomb. Many religious leaders did not respect Jesus. They wanted to be sure He didn't make good on His promise to come back to life. They had a hunch it would come true. But they didn't want it to! They had the tomb sealed. A large rock blocked it. No one could get in. And they *thought* no one could get out! Soldiers stood guard outside the tomb.

Two women who loved Jesus went to His tomb. It had been three days since His death. The ground rumbled under their feet. An angel appeared, shining bright with heaven's light.

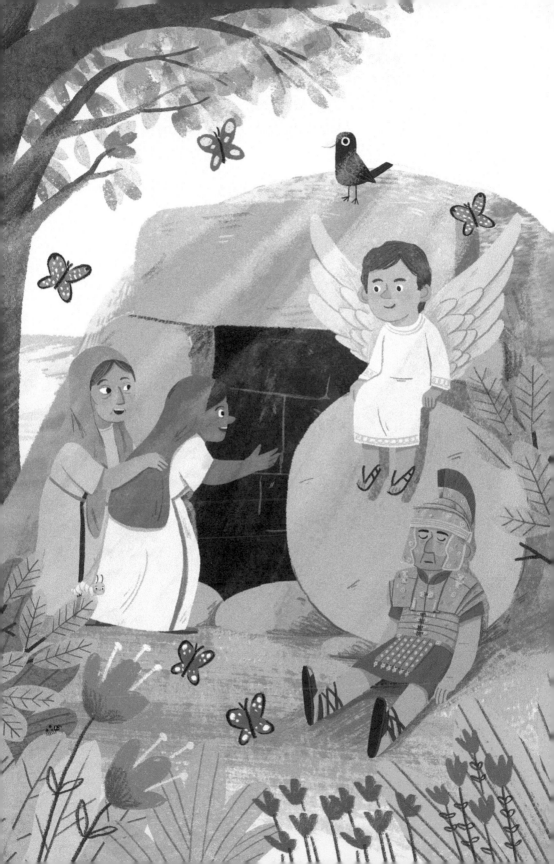

The angel rolled the giant stone away. Then he sat atop it. The guards were terrified. They fainted at the shock of it!

The angel spoke quickly to the women. He didn't want to scare them, too! "Don't be afraid," the angel said. "You are looking for Jesus, the One Who was killed on a cross. He's not here! He has risen from death, like He said He would." The angel told the women to spread the good news: *Jesus is alive!*

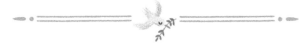

Jesus said, "All power in heaven and on earth is given to Me. You can be sure that I will be with you always. I will continue with you until the end of the world."

Matthew 28:18–20

Easter Sunday is a time for remembering all Jesus did and taught and rejoice that He lives! Jesus proves that life is everlasting! What part of the happy Easter celebration do you like best? Does your family have a favorite tradition?

JESUS RETURNS TO HEAVEN

MATTHEW 28, LUKE 24, JOHN 14

Jesus walked out of the tomb. He was very much alive! He spent time with His friends and disciples. Jesus told them things that made their hearts happy and hopeful.

"I love you. My Father loves you. I have to leave you for a little while. But you'll *never* be alone! God is sending you a best friend." Jesus was talking about the Holy Spirit. He loves all people, too! He's not seen, but He is sensed. He provides understanding of all that Jesus taught. The disciples felt joyful and sad at the same time. It would be hard to see Jesus go.

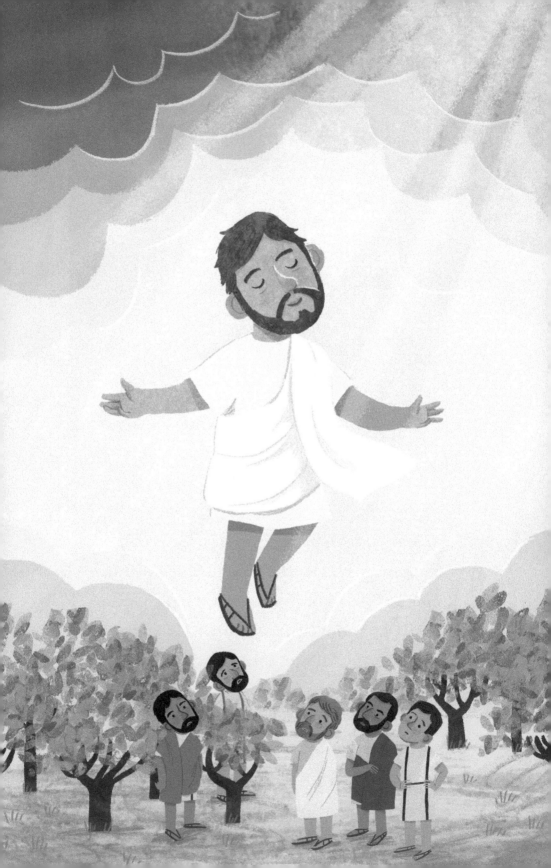

They walked with Jesus. They went to the Mount of Olives. Jesus said, "I'm going back to heaven now. I have a lot to do! I'm going to get everything ready. There will come a time when we'll be together forever. I'm coming back to this very spot one day! God will tell Me when He's ready to make all things new again."

Then, Jesus disappeared into the clouds. It was like when a balloon floats up into the air and out of sight. His followers watched Him go. They watched with wonder and excitement. They looked forward to doing what Jesus had told them to do: "Tell everyone I gave My life to make them new. I love them that much! If they believe in Me, I promise we'll be together forever."

Thomas said to Jesus, "Lord, we don't know where You are going. So how can we know the way?" Jesus answered, "I am the way. And I am the truth and the life."

John 14:5–6

❓ *The Holy Spirit lives in our hearts. God provided the Holy Spirit as a helper. How can the Holy Spirit help you today?*

SAUL HEARS THE CALL

ACTS 9

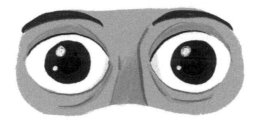

Before returning to heaven, Jesus went to His disciples. He told them to keep teaching. So the disciples taught about Jesus. They taught about the kingdom of heaven. Soon, thousands believed Jesus was God's Son. Jesus was the One who came to make hearts new again.

There was a well-known leader. His name was Saul of Tarsus. Saul didn't believe Jesus

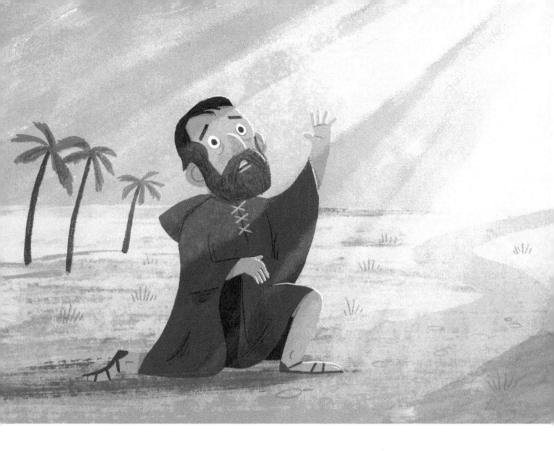

was the Savior. Saul spent all his time trying to silence those who believed in Jesus. One day, Saul was on his way to the city of Damascus. He wanted to frighten more of Jesus's believers. But God stopped Saul! A sudden bright light blasted from heaven. It knocked Saul off his feet.

A voice said, "Saul, Saul, why do you hurt Me?"

Saul asked, "Who are You, Lord?"

"I'm Jesus, the one you **persecute**! When you get to Damascus, I'll tell you what to do."

Saul was blind for three days. His eyes were closed. But his heart was open. It opened up to the love of Jesus. God restored Saul's sight. Saul was excited about serving Jesus! He became known to the world as the **apostle** Paul.

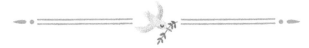

Saul began to preach about Jesus in the synagogues, saying, "Jesus is the Son of God!" All the people who heard him were amazed. They said, "This is the man who was trying to destroy those who trust in this name!"

Acts 9:19–21

❓ You have an important purpose in God's plan. What do you think God has chosen you to do? Have you asked Him for guidance? God likes to give little "winks" and "nods," so pay attention.

A HEART LIKE JESUS

ACTS 9

There was a woman named Tabitha, who loved Jesus. She wanted to be like Him. She always did good things for people. She liked to help with their needs.

Tabitha had a lot of friends. She was kind to everyone. The love of Jesus was in her heart. God wanted her to serve the poor. She made shirts and coats for people who didn't have them. Her hands were busy. She served others every day! But she became sick and died. Many people were sad. But they were also

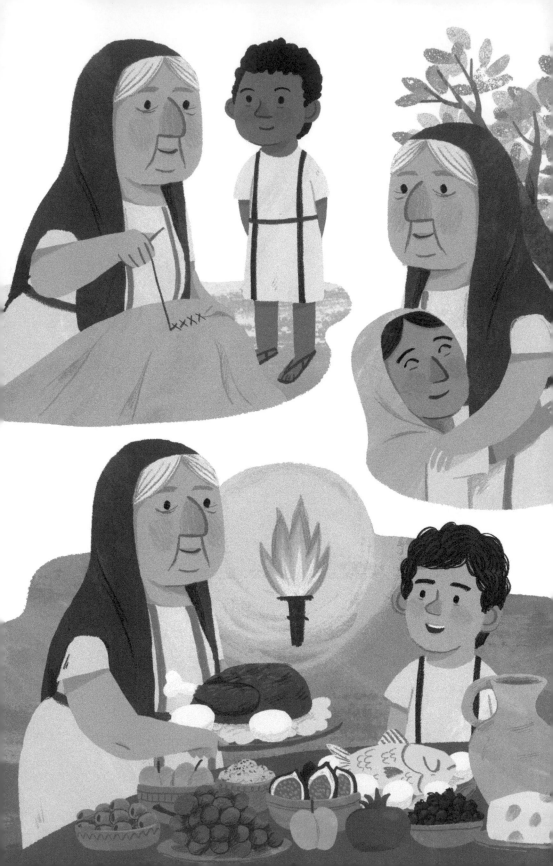

hopeful. They sent for Peter, one of Jesus's disciples. They knew Peter had done miracles, like Jesus.

Peter came to the house where Tabitha laid. The house was filled with sadness. Peter asked everyone to leave the room. He got on his knees to pray. Then Peter said, "Tabitha, get up." Her eyes opened! The house went from sadness to celebration! The people of the city heard about God's miracle. Many became followers of Jesus's teachings. His goodness had spread through Tabitha's life. She showed everyone the ever-giving love of God.

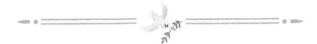

Tabitha opened her eyes, and when she saw Peter, she sat up. He gave her his hand and helped her up. Then he called the believers into the room. Tabitha was alive!

Acts 9:40–41

? *What do you enjoy doing to show the generous love of God? Sharing doesn't always involve physical items. You can share joy. You can share a kind word. You can share a song. You can share a special skill, like Tabitha did when she sewed clothing for people.*

A PRAYER TO SERVE LIKE JESUS

Dear God,

Show me how to serve with kindness, more and more each day. Make my heart like the heart of Jesus, so love comes through in every way.

A PEEK AT OUR FOREVER HOME

BOOK OF REVELATION

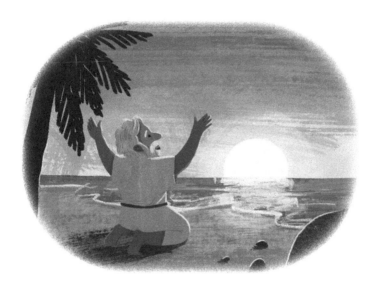

J ohn was a follower of Jesus. In his old age, John was sent away to an island by himself. He was being punished for telling people about Jesus. Then Jesus came to him saying: "I'm going to show

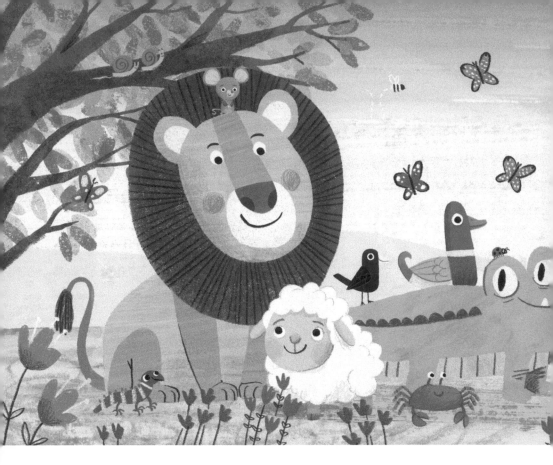

you the forever home, Heaven, that's coming. We'll live together as a family on a brand-new earth."

God wants earth to be a perfect, beautiful home for all He created. In the new home, God wipes away tears. He takes away sadness. He doesn't let *anything* hurt *anyone*. Hearts are happy all the time!

In this bright new home, Jesus is King. He rules the whole earth with kindness and love. In this perfect place, God's goodness is like a big hug that lasts *forever*.

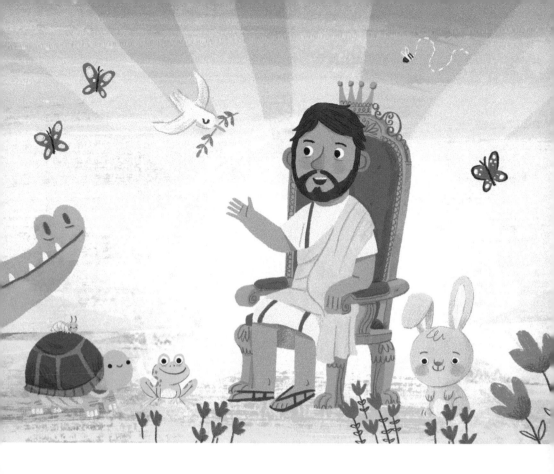

Jesus Christ is the One who loves us.
And He is the One who made us free.

Revelation 1:5

❓ *Do you know that **we** are God's favorite creation? What is your favorite part of the earthly home God created for us? Is it the ocean, the mountains, an animal, flower, or tree?*

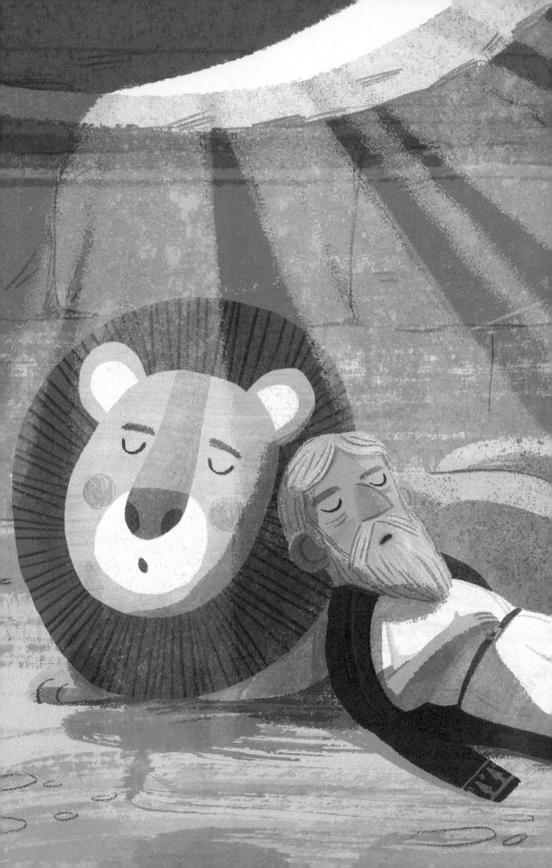

apostle: one of the twelve personal followers of Jesus during His life

ark: the ship built by Noah to save his family and two of every kind of animal

astonished: greatly surprised

awe: a feeling of wonder

comfort: lifting or lightening a person's feelings of sadness or pain

commandment: a rule given by God, such as one of the Ten Commandments

counselor: a person who guides us about how to behave

disciple: anyone who goes on to share Jesus's teachings

eternal: lasting or existing forever; without end or beginning

faith: complete trust in God without seeing proof

famine: extreme shortage of food

forgiveness: the act of letting go of bad feelings around a wrongdoing

generous: giving more of something than is expected; showing kindness to others

governor: somebody in charge of running a large community of people, such as a city or a state

holy: devoted entirely to God or the work of God

humble: to be simple, plain, or to feel less important than others

idol: an image of a god used as an object of worship

innocent: pure or blameless

joy: a feeling of great pleasure and happiness

judge: somebody who gives a fair decision on a conflict, disagreement, or situation

loyalty: the quality of being faithful or devoted

mandate: an official order to do something

miracle: a surprising and welcome event only possible with the help of God

mother-in-law: the mother of one's husband or wife (Ruth was the mother of Naomi's husband)

parable: a simple story used to illustrate a spiritual lesson

persecute: to treat someone, or a group of people, badly because of their differences from other groups

pharaoh: a ruler in ancient Egypt

prevail: to come out ahead of a challenge

promised land: the land of Canaan, which became Israel, that was promised to Abraham and his descendants

prophet: a person who speaks to people on behalf, or for, God

reign: the period during which a king or a queen rules

religious: having a belief in a god, or gods

restore: bring back; repair to its original condition

resurrection: coming back to life after death

sin: failing or refusing to follow one or more of God's rules

stature: a person's natural height and build

voyage: a long journey involving travel, usually by sea

wisdom: the quality of having knowledge and good judgment (like Deborah and King Solomon)

zither: a stringed musical instrument

AUTHOR BIO

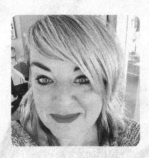

Bonnie Rickner Jensen loves to write for children and believes every child holds a unique purpose. She's a best-selling author who surrounds herself with picture books, the people she loves, and trinkets from her travels. Born in Ohio, she now calls Florida home.

ILLUSTRATOR BIO

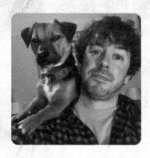

Patrick Corrigan was born in Cheshire, England. With a passion for precision as a child, he grew up patiently drawing and designing arts and crafts. Patrick worked as an art director for 10 years at a busy design studio, where he contributed to more than 500 educational and picture books for children. He is now based in Hammersmith, West London, where he lives with his newspaper editor wife, Dulcie, and their fat cat, Forbes.

CPSIA information can be obtained
at www.ICGtesting.com
Printed in the USA
JSHW022034130621
15838JS00002B/2